Everyday
Voice Care

Everyday Voice Care

The Lifestyle Guide for
Singers and Talkers

Joanna Cazden

Hal Leonard Books
An Imprint of Hal Leonard Corporation

Published in 2012
An Imprint of Hal Leonard Corporation
7777 West Bluemound Road
Milwaukee, WI 53213

Trade Book Division Editorial Offices
33 Plymouth St., Montclair, NJ 07042

Printed in the United States of America

Book design by Leslie Goldman
Illustrations by Joanna Cazden
Cover photograph from Shutterstock

Library of Congress Cataloging-in-Publication Data

Cazden, Joanna.
Everyday voice care : the lifestyle guide for singers and talkers / Joanna Cazden.
pages cm
Includes bibliographical references.
1. Voice–Care and hygiene 2. Voice culture. 3. Voice–Physiological aspects. I. Title.
MT821.C35 2012
612.7'8–dc23
2012025310

ISBN 978-1-4584-4318-2

www.halleonardbooks.com

To human voices everywhere:
known or unknown, celebrated or silenced,
pristine or damaged, fluent or tentative,
those no longer with us
and those voices yet to be heard.

Contents

Acknowledgments

I have learned from so many people over so many years that it is certain some will be overlooked. Here, therefore, is an assuredly partial list of those who have helped me understand the voice and its care, and those who helped this book to exist. None carry any blame for my errors.

Thanks to my first voice teachers: Kitty Miller, Ellalou "Pete" Dimmock, and choral master Thomas Vasil, for a safe, healthy start. To the theater and theater-voice faculties of the University of Washington, American Conservatory Theater, and CalArts, for their liberating disciplines of voice, speech, mind, and body. To the faculty and staff in Communication Disorders and Sciences, California State University, Northridge, for training, encouragement, and teaching opportunities. To clinical mentors Judith Trost-Cardamone, Nancy Sedat, Carol Kyser Scott, Linda Gasson, and Sherry Washington, for their exemplary intelligence, discipline, ethics, and compassion. To cross-disciplinary pioneers Katherine Verdolini Abbott and Lucille Rubin for encouraging my ventures. And to the ongoing wisdom of the American Speech-Language and Hearing Association's Special Interest Group in Voice Disorders.

Thanks to my current voice teacher and mentor Catherine Fitzmaurice for profound retraining. Thanks to the community of Fitzmaurice "Trems" and my many friends and colleagues in the Voice and Speech Trainers Association for keeping me grounded, warmed, and inspired.

Thanks to the laryngologists at Cedars-Sinai Medical Center and elsewhere who have shared their knowledge and trusted me with their patients: especially Drs. David Alessi, Robert Andrews, Michel Babajanian, Gary Bellack, Mark Courey, Steven Feinberg, Matthew Finerman, Reena Gupta, Garrett Herzon, Martin Hopp, Babak Larian, Warren Line, Rafi Mesrobian, Madison Richardson, Robert Sataloff, Hans Von Leden, and Mani Zadeh. Thanks also to my patients and students for ongoing reminders of what's important in the human condition.

Thanks to the following for permission to quote from their websites: Alexander Massey (www.oxfordsinginglessons.co.uk) and Ray Sahelian, MD (www.raysahelian.com). Thanks to Ron Stone for permission to use his posts to the vocal-health forum The Modern Vocalist World (www.themodernvocalist.com), and thanks to Elissa Weinzimmer for her diligent research on throat lozenges.

Exceptional thanks to Scott Wilkinson, my partner in life, music, science, and writing, for loving companionship and many rounds of editing.

Thanks above all to the Source of All Creation, who keeps us in life, who sustains us, and who brings us to this present moment.

I

Foundation:
About Your Voice

If all my possessions were taken from me with one exception,
I would choose to keep the power of communication, for by
it I would soon regain all the rest.
—Daniel Webster

A defective voice will always preclude an artist from
achieving the complete development of his art, however
intelligent he may be. . . . The voice is an instrument
which the artist must learn to use with suppleness and
sureness, as if it were a limb.
—Sarah Bernhardt

It is through our desires, our sensations, our perceptions,
that we gain control of our activities in body and mind.
This is especially true in singing. A friend, a book,
a word, a look may help or harm us. We find by
experience what is hurtful or helpful.
—Giovanni Battista Lamperti

1

Consciousness and Contradictions

There is much music, excellent voice, in this little organ.
—From *Hamlet*, by William Shakespeare

Anything anyone might say on the subject of the human voice would be at variance with the opinions of others. There is probably no subject in human ken in which there is such a marked difference of opinion.
—Evan Williams

The voice, as an instrument of sound and speech, has historically been difficult to study and understand. It is small, is out of sight inside the throat, moves quickly, and much of what it does is unconscious.

Located right where we breathe and swallow, the vocal mechanism is shielded by survival reflexes. Although we use it to extend thoughts and feelings outside of ourselves, toward others, many aspects of vocal function are more deeply internal than our normal awareness, more similar to the visceral organs than to the familiar workings of the mouth.

The muscles and surfaces of the voice box don't have the same kinds of sensors that the limbs, hands, and tongue do. Sensations are not clear; feelings of discomfort in the voice are often vague, not localized. What we feel, or what we think we feel, in the throat and in our voices is not always reliable information about what is happening inside.

Fast Vibration

This small vocal organ is not only out of sight and disconnected from conscious experience, but its functions are also hidden by the element of time, for they are too fast for the naked eye to grasp.

The first known observation of the vocal cords in motion was in 1854, by an Italian singing teacher named Manuel Garcia, using a little mirror and a candle. At best, he would have seen a small triangular valve with indistinctly buzzing edges.

The little muscles that put the vocal cords into position to vibrate are held relatively steady during modern laryngeal exams, as long or short tones are cued by the examiner. But in the normal flow of speech, the vocal on/off switch flickers from 10 to 15 times per second to create the vowels, consonants, inhalations, and microtimed pauses of each language.

Once set in motion by the airstream, the vocal cords themselves vibrate from as few as 50 to over 1,000 times per second—far too fast to be observed and understood until the optical technologies of the past decades. So the entire subject has been mysterious for a long time, and it is no one's fault.

Detailed visual study of the voice in action came much later, because it required film cameras and light sources small enough and flexible enough to reach inside the throat without gagging or choking the person who was awake and making sound. Eventually, strobe-light technology brought a virtual slow-motion view that began to reveal the vibratory movements of the vocal cords; this is now extended by ultra-high-speed research cameras. Meanwhile, microscopic views of the vocal folds in cross-section have revealed multiple layers and gel-like qualities that help to explain how the cords vibrate, stretch, and react to being bruised.

In the 21st century, fiber-optic (analog) laryngoscopes are gradually being replaced by digital systems. These visual tools are complemented by digital analysis of vocally produced sound waves and by other advanced sensors of air pressure, muscle activity, and nerve conduction. Nevertheless, much remains unknown.

Science Versus History

In the medical literature, the vocal cord is a mere fold, a piece of gristle that strives to reach out and touch its twin, thus producing the possibility of sound effects.
But I feel that there must be a deep relationship with the word "chord": the resonant vibration that can stir memory, produce music, evoke love, bring tears, move crowds to pity and mobs to passion.
—Christopher Hitchens

In almost all cultures, at the creation the Gods gave the people songs.
—Clarissa Pinkola Estés

In contrast to the young, technology-dependent fields of voice science and medicine, the interpersonal and cultural uses of voice are as old as human society. Vocal sound provides the foundation of speech, one of our most basic ways to share information and feelings with other people.

Communities or tribes also rely on vocal sound to express group identity—through music, religion, poetry, storytelling, bardic recitations of history, work songs, children's games, and magic incantations. The nuances of voice, and how we choose and sequence throat-and-mouth sounds into complex communication, are close to the core of civilization itself and to our nature as social human beings.

Curiosity about this vital instrument is understandable, as are the traditional healing practices and home remedies that have evolved to manage a thousand generations of hoarseness and sore throats. Speculation and guesswork about the voice and its care may be as old, and as close to our ancestral memories, as voice use itself.

But without the ability to know for sure, beliefs about vocal function and health have been as often wrong as the belief that the sun travels around the earth, or that women determine the sex of their children. Meanwhile our science-based understanding of the voice is hundreds of years younger than Copernicus, decades newer than the genetics of gender.

All in all, our current situation can be seen as perhaps 50 years of science crashing into 50,000 years of folklore, the latter often closer than the former to each individual's everyday experience of their own voice. Many scientific facts don't match internal sensation or cultural practice, so it's no surprise that popular misunderstandings have lasted so long.

It all adds up to an exciting time to work in the field of voice, and a complicated time for everyone involved. Every vocal artist's inner sense is partly right and partly wrong. Conferences on vocal science, medicine, and the processes of teaching voice are crammed with many more questions than answers.

The explanations in this book are drawn from my experience with hundreds of medical patients and vocal-arts students as well as my own journeys as an artist, teacher, therapist, and clinical educator. I've learned what voice patients tend to disbelieve about their hoarseness, and I honor the individual, internal experience of the voice even when it doesn't match objective fact.

I also recognize that our experiences of the body and of health-care practice are themselves influenced by culture, environment, and economic resources. No specific instructions or voice-care recipe will fit every reader's circumstances. I hope that the principles offered here are clear enough that if my suggestions don't fit your life, you can invent something better.

More than anything, I know that each voice is unique, and your voice is your own—physiologically, vocationally, and spiritually. You're reading this book because you want to be a healthier, better-informed voice user. The next chapters will provide what you need to get started.

Chapter 1 Summary

- The voice as a physical organ has been hard to understand until recent decades.

- It is hard to see, hard to feel, hard to investigate, and hard to ignore.

- Scientific knowledge about the voice is as new as folk beliefs about it are old.

- Sensations and feelings about voice may not fit the emerging objective information.

- Understanding and tolerating that contradiction is part of the health journey of every serious voice user.

2

How the Voice Works

*The voice collects and translates your bad physical health,
your emotional worries, your personal troubles.*
—Placido Domingo

I f you want to take good care of your voice, start by understanding how it works. The voice box, medically called the *larynx* (pronounced "<u>laa</u>-rinks," not "<u>lahr</u>-niks"), is a complicated framework of cartilage, about the size of a walnut. Its most visible landmark is the point of the Adam's apple in your throat.

The larynx is considered part of the respiratory system. It sits on top of the windpipe (*trachea*), the passage to your lungs, and directly in front of the top valve of your digestive tube (*esophagus*), as shown in **Fig. 1**. So the vocal mechanism is located at an important spot in the body in terms of basic survival—the point of divergence between eating and breathing.

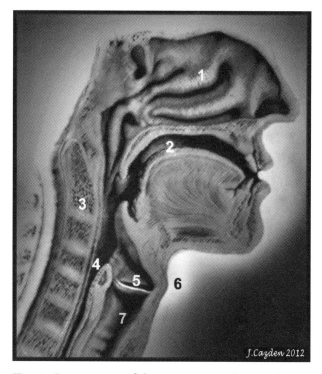

Fig. 1: Cutaway view of the upper airway showing the position of one vocal fold inside the larynx and related structures, including (1) nose, (2) mouth, (3) cervical vertebrae, (4) esophagus = path to stomach, (5) vocal fold, (6) point of Adam's apple, and (7) trachea = path to lungs.

How the Voice Is Built

Two small folds of flexible tissue run from front to back inside the larynx. These vocal folds—more commonly called the vocal "cords" or sometimes the vocal "bands"—are about one centimeter long. (Throughout this book, I will use the words "cords" and "folds" interchangeably, preferring the word "cords" because it is more common in nonprofessional settings.)

In the typical exam view, looking down from behind your tongue (see **Fig. 2**), these look like neither stringy cords nor repeated folds, but like two little shelves arranged in a V shape. The point of the V is at the front, directly behind the Adam's apple (a cartilage landmark that exists in children and women but with a shallower, less prominent angle than in postpuberty men).

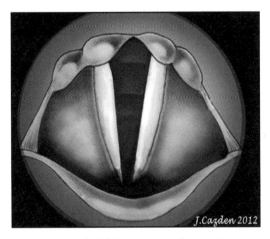

Fig. 2: Vocal folds as seen from above, in normal position for quiet breathing.

The vocal folds are made of small muscles, covered first with a slightly stiff, gel-like substance, and then with a very loose, moist mucous membrane (also called the *mucosa*). A whitish ligament—again, about 1 cm long—stiffens each of the two vibrating edges, a bit like a thick hem protecting the edge of a fabric or a curtain rod stabilizing the more fluid curtain.

The soft, wet outermost layer is just like the lining inside your mouth. It coats the entire throat, through the larynx, until it merges down into the lining of the trachea and the bronchial tubes that branch into your lungs. Most of the larynx is the same pink color as your throat, indicating a dense blood supply. Where the mucous layer covers the whiter ligament at the edge, the healthy vocal fold looks pale, milky white.

Online, you can now find lots of pictures and videos taken with a strobe light that show how the vocal folds move. Just as with noses and hands, each person's larynx has slightly different proportions and characteristics. Yours is unique, and your vocal cords interact with your personality and language to create a vocal sound that is entirely your own.

How Your Vocal Cords Move

In general, the larynx helps to regulate the flow of air in and out of the body. Along the way, it can also turn airflow into sound.

At the front of the larynx, right behind the Adam's apple, the two vocal folds are attached next to each other, making the front corner of the V shape. At the back, the folds attach separately to smaller bits of cartilage that can pivot toward or away from each other. Like a flexible valve in the middle of a plumbing pipe or swinging double doors in a restaurant kitchen, the position of the vocal folds affects the flow of air in and out of the body.

When the vocal folds pivot apart, a triangular space appears between them; this space is called the *glottis*. It is an important doorway, and whether open or closed, is an important boundary. In the medical world, everything that relates to breathing above the level of the vocal cords or glottis is grouped together as the "upper respiratory tract"; everything below the glottis is the "lower respiratory tract." As the structures of the larynx thus serve as the "final gate" of protection for the lungs, the voice exists exactly between the consciously movable mouth and throat, and the unconscious, life-preserving visceral organs.

When you take in a deep breath, for instance during heavy exercise or when you savor the smell of a favorite food or perfume, the vocal folds are farthest apart. The glottis is wide open and there's a free passage between the lungs and the upper airway.

When the lungs need protection, the vocal folds squeeze together to close the glottis. This happens reflexively every time you swallow.

Other reflexes can flicker the glottis open and closed, creating shifts in air pressure and flow that help to clean the airway. The vocal folds clap together briefly to "clear your throat," and they bang together more vigorously in the cough that expels phlegm, smoke, or dust that your lungs need to get rid of.

How Your Voice Makes Sound

Between the two extremes of being far apart and closed tightly together, the vocal folds can close partway, reducing the breath stream without completely stopping it. For a normal vocal sound, the vocal folds move to a position where their edges just barely touch.

Small support muscles interact with the vocal-fold muscles themselves, creating the right elastic tension for the loudness and pitch you want to produce. Then, when a constant, smooth stream of air from the lungs flows out between the vocal folds, they vibrate and make an audible tone. This act of producing sound, coordinating the vocal muscles with the flow of breath, is formally called *phonation,* from the Greek root *phon,* which means *sound.*

If the vocal folds are close to each other, partially blocking the

airway but not in the exact position to vibrate, they simply create turbulence in the air. The result is a whooshing, breathy sound known
as a whisper.

A set of specialized muscles at the front of the larynx stretch the
vocal folds longer and thinner (for a higher pitch) or let them get
short and thick (for a lower pitch), much like a rubber band. Sometimes the muscle layer disengages, but the softer layers still vibrate;
this is called "falsetto" or "head voice."

All of these adjustments, combined with changes in the breath
stream that sets the cords in motion, create vocal loudness, pitch,
inflection, and emotional tone. Problems can arise at any level, from
the health of laryngeal cells to the demands of a public community.

While some disruptions to the larynx are beyond your control,
simple health habits can go a long way toward keeping your voice in
working order. You can skip ahead to those guidelines, or follow me
through a little more theory about how the voice develops and how it
can get into trouble.

Chapter 2 Summary

- The vocal folds (cords) are small, mobile, and muscular, located inside a protective frame of cartilage called the larynx.

- The vocal cords work as a valve, opening and closing your airway at a special place called the glottis.

- The larynx and the vocal cords inside it regulate breathing and contribute to familiar reflexes such as coughing or closing the airway when you swallow.

- The sound of the voice is created when the vocal folds are closed in just the right position and set in motion by the right kind of airflow. These actions are only partly conscious.

- Although vocal function is complicated, keeping it healthy can be quite simple.

3

How Voices Grow and Why They Suffer

Speech is the means by which the soul expresses itself.
—Galen

*For my voice, I have lost it with halloing
and singing of anthems.*
—From *King Henry IV, Part II*, by William Shakespeare

When a baby is born, everyone waits for the first cry, announcing that this new person has a functioning airway. Individual survival and communication emerge at the same instant.

Obviously, raw phonation is natural and needs no special training. But a baby isn't able to control the muscles of its breath, voice, throat, and mouth in order to make specific sounds. Indeed, the word "infant" in Latin literally means "the speechless one."

Vocal skills begin to develop within the first few months of life. Babies typically spend many hours babbling, exploring a wide variety of cries, sighs, consonants, and melodics. Through this early vocal play, our brains learn how to control the position, length, thickness, and internal tension of the vocal folds.

A normal toddler doesn't consciously know how those controls work when he or she is talking. It just happens. We learn that different sounds have different effects on the people around us. We notice that older people manipulate sound inside their mouths.

We practice shaping the vibrations and airflow into vowels and consonants. Communicating with more skillful sounds, and then with words, helps us get our needs met and express ourselves. In early childhood, as our speech becomes more complex, we rely on our voices to carry messages of what we want and how we feel, as well as to comment on or ask about things and events around us.

We copy the melody of the language spoken around us, its resonance and inflection. We learn to create a loud voice for some situations and a very quiet sound for others. Invisibly, and usually unconsciously, the larynx and breath mechanism become skilled at all these variations.

Both girls' and boys' voices change during adolescence, although the growth and pointed shape of the developing male larynx are the more dramatic. As we mature into adulthood, each individual's muscle habits, the size and shape of their throat, and the power of their breath combine with personality, life experience, and education to produce a vocal sound that is as unique as a fingerprint.

Those of us who use our voices in public learn to do so with even more precision, range, power, efficiency, and nuance. When the larynx and breathing mechanisms work together effectively, our loudness, phrasing, pitch inflection, and tone of voice perfectly carry the meaning of what we think and how we feel.

Why Good Voices Go Bad

I don't ever recall speculating much about being struck dumb. . . . Deprivation of the ability to speak is more like an attack of impotence, or the amputation of part of the personality.

—Christopher Hitchens

Under normal circumstances, the voice serves many wonderful purposes, automatically and unconsciously. It is therefore easy to take your voice for granted until something goes wrong.

If your larynx and vocal technique are healthy, you express yourself easily, with no feeling of effort or even of use. But when the vocal mechanism stops working correctly, or you're pushing beyond your abilities, you probably won't get a clear, detailed message or warning.

Hoarseness is not as specific as the feeling of a stubbed toe, skinned knee, or toothache. Instead, the vocal cords get your attention with vague discomfort, husky sound, or glitchy sensations. You might start to notice a tickle, a cough, a general feeling

It's Not Supposed to Hurt

I taught myself to sing and write songs, and some producers got interested, so my family moved to Hollywood. My throat hurt all the time, but I thought it was normal, so I didn't tell anyone.

I didn't want vocal lessons because I thought they would keep me from sounding natural. But finally I talked to my mom, and she said that maybe my throat shouldn't be hurting.

It took a year for me to agree to go to the doctor, get some help and training. Now I'm so glad I did. Singing doesn't hurt anymore, and I still sound like I want to. Better, actually.

—a student

of tension or effort, a vague ache.

Sometimes only the sound will change, while the feel of the mechanism stays normal. Or it can be the other way around. Signs that your voice isn't functioning as it should: talking or singing is tiring, it's harder to be very soft or very loud, you experience throat pain or tickling or some other discomfort that doesn't go away, or getting the sound you want just takes more work than it used to.

How do changes in the vocal cells make you hoarse? With overuse or injury, the vibrating edges of the vocal folds can become bruised, swollen, or scarred. If they can't form a clean seal when they touch, closure of the glottis is irregular or incomplete. The cords don't vibrate evenly, extra air leaks through the gaps, and the voice sounds rough.

Other health or usage problems can make the vocal folds paralyzed, stiff, weak, or jumpy. The larynx can be taken over by fungal infections, stubborn viruses, or by cancer, any of which change the sound and/or sensations of the voice or breathing in a variety of ways.

Diseases that affect the nervous system, air supply, fluid balance, or other aspects of general health can also get in the way of good vocal function. The larynx can be bruised by direct injuries to the throat, such as from an accidental elbow jab during sports or from hitting a steering wheel during a car accident.

Treatment of unrelated problems can also result in unfortunate vocal side effects. This "collateral damage" to the voice can follow surgeries to the heart, neck, or thyroid gland as well as radiation treatments to the neck, mouth, or face.

The good news is that most voice problems are caused simply by how—and how much—the voice is being used, exacerbated by common respiratory or digestive conditions. Most voice problems are also relatively simple to treat, especially if you can get help from the small-but-growing community of medical and rehabilitation professionals who specialize in voice treatment.

If most problems are simple, why write so many chapters? Because the purpose of this book is to *prevent* problems, and that can require attention to many different aspects of your lifestyle, everyday habits, communication environment, and attitude.

The suggestions in this book will help you keep your voice healthy, get the right kind of help when you need it, and recover when trouble strikes. Once you understand the principles, you can find—and invent—more answers on your own.

Chapter 3 Summary

- Normal vocal function is automatic; we don't feel much until something goes wrong.

- Vocal skills develop along with the other aspects of speech and self-expression, maturing at the crossroads of our bodies and our place in society.

- The vocal cords react to overuse, illness, physical injury, and medical conditions that show up elsewhere in the body.

- Changes in how your voice sounds and feels are signals that something in your life, health, or voice technique needs attention.

- It is normal for these changes to appear by surprise and to carry the experience of a profound personal loss.

- The focus of this book is on preventing the simplest, most common voice problems. It will also help you work with a voice doctor (laryngologist) when prevention and home remedies aren't enough.

4

Quick Rules for Vocal Wellness

- **Vocal cords have needs and limits.** They are powerful and flexible for their size, vulnerable to a variety of irritants, and swift to recover when given the chance. They work better with care and training.

- **Vocal cords like moisture.** They work better when the body is internally hydrated and the air is somewhat humid. Dry vocal cords in a dehydrated body will get tired and rough very fast.

- **Vocal cords need rest.** They benefit from small rest breaks here and there, and longer stretches of silence after heavy use. Even five minutes of rest helps the vocal cells recover from the pressure and vibrations of speech.

- **Vocal cords like variety.** Use a wide inflection range as you talk. Simply adding animation to your voice—a little bit of the energy you use when talking to children or pets—makes it easier for others to listen, and it gives your vocal cords more changes of position, more chances to stretch and relax.

- **Your voice reflects your overall health and vitality.** Many aspects of health and wellness indirectly impact your voice. So everything you do to take care of yourself also helps you sound great.

Keeping your body healthy is an expression of gratitude to the whole cosmos—the trees, the clouds, everything.
—Thich Nhat Hanh

Chapter 4 Summary

- Respect your vocal cords and learn how to give them good care.

- Pay special attention to humidity and hydration. For details, see chapter 5, "Air" and chapter 7, "Drink."

- Know when to stop vocalizing, as explained in chapter 8, "Voice Rest."

- Protect the vocal muscles and surfaces with flexible, comfortable use. Learn more in Chapter 9, "Warming Up the Voice," and chapter 23, "Training."

II

Prevention:
Basic Voice Care

Blest be the man who first invented sleep—a cloak to
cover all human imaginings, food to satisfy hunger, water
to quench thirst, fire to warm cold air, cold to temper heat,
and lastly, a coin to buy whatever we need.
—Miguel Cervantes

If we could give every individual the right amount of
nourishment and exercise, not too little and not too much,
we would have found the safest way to health.
—Hippocrates

It is hardly necessary to remind the student that
without nutritious food and warm clothing
the voice will not endure.
—Manuel Garcia

Nothing so needs reforming as other people's habits.
—Mark Twain

5

Air

Sound is naught but broken air: and every speech
that is uttered, aloud or privily, good or ill, is in
substance nothing but air.

—**Geoffrey Chaucer**

An inspiration is an idea and a breath—I'm breathing in
because I have something that I want to express to you.

—**Catherine Fitzmaurice**

The vocal folds vibrate in response to a stream of air flowing out of the body. The voice box and the breathing areas above it (the upper respiratory tract) also filter the air coming into the body. The quality of air coming in affects the health of the entire area.

Both your nose and your mouth—the entry passages for air— are lined with moist mucous membranes. Air passing through these passages picks up moisture and begins to match the inner body temperature. While the mouth is a large, simple opening, the nose is a curly "obstacle course," allowing a more prolonged effect on environmental air.

The nasal membranes also contain thousands of microscopic hairs (*cilia*) whose job is to catch dust, allergens, and anything else that could hurt your lungs. By the time air gets to the voice box, it is warm, humid, and filtered.

If these entry passages are overly dry—because the nose is congested and one breathes only through the mouth, or perhaps because medication or whole-body dehydration have decreased fluid levels between cells—the larynx will also become dry.

Other airborne problems for the voice come in the form of irritating chemicals, extreme temperatures, or infectious bugs that the nose and mouth didn't catch. The most common, controllable irritant is cigarette smoke, discussed at length in chapter 22, "Tobacco, Alcohol, and Marijuana."

General air pollution hurts the lungs and can trigger allergic reactions throughout the airway. Unless these reactions lead to chronic allergic inflammation, a chronic cough, or severe asthmatic conditions that restrict breath use for speech, I haven't seen a direct link between pollution and the voice.

Should I Breathe Through My Nose or My Mouth?

I'm often asked this question. It's one of many subjects about which I recommend flexible common sense rather than an absolute rule.

Breathing through the nose allows for the filtering I've just described, and it may be subtly more relaxing to the nervous system. Some singing teachers emphasize inhaling through the nose as a way of opening the upper throat for an improved sense of resonance.

Using nose and mouth together obviously helps to take in a larger amount of air, and this is definitely needed during exercise, dance, or other physical exertion.

But your nasal passages might be anatomically small, congested (swollen) from allergies or illness, or partially clogged by dust or other debris. So don't waste energy or anxiety about whether it is "wrong" to breathe through your mouth.

Air is important enough to your survival that your body has more than one passageway. Your unconscious systems will use what works best in a given situation with the instrument you have. If nose breathing isn't possible for you on a given day, just take extra care to get enough moisture into the air, as described in the next section.

> Breath occupies the most active place in human vocal production. It is the energy impulse that excites the vibration in the vocal folds and the resulting resonance in the body—starting, continuing, and stopping it.
> —Catharine Fitzmaurice

Moisturizing the Airway

In chapter 7, "Drink," I discuss water as a beverage. But humidity in the air you breathe is also important to keep the surfaces of the larynx comfortable.

In humid climates, this is no problem. In dry climates or environments with air-conditioning or central heat, your voice will be happier if you add moisture. Many clients tell me their voices feel and sound better in Hawaii or Florida than in Los Angeles! In general, if you're in an area where your lips and skin tend to get dry, the lining of your airway will be dry as well.

There are many ways to increase humidity and soothe your voice with moisture. Take extralong showers when your voice is under stress and at night after a long day of talking or singing. If you have access to a steam room at your gym, health club, or apartment building, use it. (Dry saunas have other health and relaxation benefits, and short periods of use will not harm your vocal cords if you drink plenty of water before, during, and after. But if you're otherwise in an overly dry environment, choose the steam.)

Inexpensive steam appliances called "facial spas" or "facial steam spas" work very well for the voice. Some performers travel with one in their luggage. Use it daily or whenever you feel the need for extra vocal care (between rehearsal and performance, before doing your hair and makeup, can be a great time).

For the least costly home version of this type of voice care, just heat a pot of hot water, take it off the stove, and inhale from it with a towel over your head. Stay far enough above the hot water so that you don't feel any burning on your face. And of course be sure that pets or small children don't spill it by mistake.

In addition to these direct steam treatments, more diffuse humidity can be very helpful, such as from a humidifier or vaporizer next to your bed. It should be filled with water only, not commercial mentholated additives or aromatherapy oils.

A musical theater performer recently told me that he is only allowed two suitcases on tour. If he can't fit his facial steamer in his personal luggage, he packs it alongside his makeup kit, props, and other backstage gear. This extra freight allowance is now written into his contracts.

Your doctor may advise a cool-air or warm-air device. Either will serve the purpose of moisturizing the vocal folds. To avoid mold contamination, keep the device clean by following the manufacturer's instructions.

Be creative, especially if you are concerned about cost. One summer in Los Angeles, I worked with a singer who complained that her mouth and throat often felt dry in the mornings.Her apartment had no air-conditioning, and she could sleep in the hot weather only with a fan blowing close to the bed. After we talked about the importance of a humid airway, she put a bowl of water in front of the fan. Like wind carrying humid weather, the fan blew enough moisture over her face at night, that she was soon free of that morning discomfort.

Here is another humidification trick for those moments when you're in the middle of a vocal performance or presentation and your throat is drying out: Lift the tip of your tongue as if you were saying "L." This maneuver offers more wet surface area to incoming air.

If you're in the middle of a performance and your throat feels dry, return to this "L" position whenever you have a moment to rest between phrases, or between songs. Sip water too, of course. Even a few breaths this way can temporarily ease a dry throat, and no one will know.

Just as our soul, which is air, holds us together, so do breath and air encompass the whole world.
—Anaximenes

Airway Allergies

Respiratory allergies occur when the immune system overreacts to substances encountered in the airway. You may be more affected at certain times of the year or in specific environments. These sensitivities typically begin in childhood or on relocation to a new city.

Many general wellness practices, as emphasized throughout this book, can make a surprising difference in nasal congestion. A friend of mine constantly blew his nose, sniffled and sneezed, and—worst of all for his wife—snored loudly. He decided for other reasons to make some changes in diet, exercise, and how he coped with family stress. Within a year, the extra phlegm was gone, as was the snoring.

In addition to learning how to avoid the things that trigger allergies and strengthening your whole system to be less sensitive, many vocal performers use air filters or

A Cautionary Tale

Once upon a time, a singing student from overseas carefully saved enough money to travel, attend music school in the USA, and study with a particular teacher about whom she had read online. This student suffered from an allergy to cats. She could not have known, while preparing for her journey, that the teacher who ran the school always kept cats in his vocal studio. This teacher required all beginning students to work with him.

Week after week, the student went to her singing lessons, always leaving the studio with watery, itchy eyes and extra phlegm in her nose and throat. She would cough for days afterward, and within a couple of months, she became totally unable to breathe through her nose. Her voice gradually became hoarse, and she lost her highest notes.

purifiers at home as a precaution. I don't recommend any particular type of air purifier, but just as with your vaporizer or humidifier, keep it clean.

Sinus Problems

Sinuses are air-filled cavities inside the facial bones. They are lined with mucous membrane and have drainage tubes that go into the upper nose. As long as these tiny tubes stay open, extra material can drain out and bacteria-killing oxygen can seep in, maintaining a healthy chemical environment.

If the tubes become blocked—by swelling in the nose area, such as from a cold, or by mucous secretions that are too thick—the sinuses build up pressure and are more vulnerable to infection. The respiratory sinuses can also become chemically imbalanced if the mucous linings are too dry. Respiratory allergies, viruses, smoking, and many other factors contribute to problems in this region.

For short-term discomfort in the sinus area, keep the mucous

She asked to take her private lessons in a different building, away from the cats, but was refused. If she dropped any of her classes, she would lose her student visa. She had sacrificed a lot for her training, and she was miserable.

After a few months, the student was diagnosed with vocal nodules (callouses), probably due to the vigorous coughing brought on by these allergies. Only then did the school director take her concerns seriously. She was allowed to take lessons with another singing teacher.

It took about six months for this young artist to get back her full range and her pleasure in singing. If a teacher does not understand or respect vocal health, how can he or she be trusted to train healthy singing?

thin by drinking plenty of fluids; soak a washcloth in hot water, wring it out, and press to your upper face a few times per day; and inhale steam (carefully) as previously described.

Sinus and allergy reactions worsen when you are under stress. Correspondingly, the general wellness habits emphasized throughout this book (nutrition, sleep, exercise, and so on) will help your body cope with temporary irritants.

> Breathing is the bridge between mind and body, the connection between consciousness and unconsciousness, the movement of spirit in matter.
> **—Andrew Weil, MD**

Nasal Irrigation

Rinsing the nasal passages with salt water is a traditional practice in yoga that has become popular in wider communities, and many vocalists and ENT doctors favor it. This practice clears "gunk" from the back of the nose, helping the sinuses to drain normally and stay healthy.

Some vocalists perform nasal irrigation every day in their normal bathing routine. Others consider it an extra precaution during cold-and-flu season or at the first sign of a cold. If you are often congested or tend to get sinus infections, you may wish to use nasal irrigation regularly.

Irrigation appliances direct a stream of water into your nose, similar to a dental "water pick" but with less pressure. Saline sprays and squirt bottles are milder, portable variations on the same theme, easily found over the counter at drugstores.

A small cup with a long spout, called a Neti pot in the yoga tradi-tion of Ayurvedic medicine, does the same job and has become popu-lar alongside other yoga practices. These are now available online and in many health-food stores and pharmacies.

When using irrigation devices, the normal recipe calls for warm water with a small amount of salt. Salt packets may be prepackaged for this use including a little baking soda (sodium bicarbonate) too, or you can mix in your own.

Here are a few suggestions on this practice from my own experi-ence, from clients, and from online forums:

- If you make your own saltwater solution, use noniodized salt! Iodized salt will sting the inside of your nose.

- The flow need not go in one nostril and out the other, as described in some Neti instructions and traditional yoga writings. The salt water can just trickle from one nostril down into your mouth and be spit out. Cleanse each nostril a few times, then gargle with any remaining liquid.

- There's some evidence that rinsing or irrigating the nose too often removes helpful secretions, overdrying and ir-ritating the nasal linings. This would increase rather than decrease the risk of infection. So for general preventative care, it may be better to rinse your nose—two to three times per week, rather than every day.

- If you like the concept of cleansing your nose but dislike the actual process, try doing it in the shower.

As always, talk to your doctor about any questions or concerns you have.

Salt Air

There is new evidence that simply breathing the air in a salty environment can help sinus, asthma, and other respiratory problems. A few high-end spa retreats now have "salt inhalation" rooms, mimicking the (less elegant) environment of underground salt mines. Commercial gadgets that allow you to breath salty air have been featured on TV health programs.

There's not enough evidence yet to clarify whether this practice is truly beneficial and for whom. It doesn't appear to be risky, though, so perhaps it's worth a try for people with chronic breathing problems.

Beyond Home Remedies

If you have chronic problems with your nose or sinuses, of course, consult with an ear-nose-throat doctor. Healthy airways are important for your vocal goals, and a low-level, chronic infection in the upper airway can contribute to laryngeal inflammation. Just be sure that the doctor understands your voice concerns and that you discuss medications and doses in order to decongest the nose without overly drying the larynx.

If nasal or sinus surgery is recommended, there is little risk of vocal problems as a result. However, changes in the internal structures of your nose and face can change your experience of vocal resonance (the sound-enriching vibrations that feel amplified in your face and head). So your voice may sound or feel different to you, more disorienting than any change in how you sound to other people. These new sensations of sound and resonance may not stabilize for several weeks.

A good voice teacher or speech pathologist can help rebalance your sound, but I've rarely been asked for this help. Of clients who have undergone some kind of sinus or nose procedure, most like their voices better afterward.

Chapter 5 Summary

- The vocal cords and the rest of your lower airway are healthiest in an environment that is clean, smoke-free, and has about 50 percent humidity.

- Steam treatments, humidifiers, and vaporizers offer important protection and "first aid" for your voice.

- Respiratory allergies and chronic sinus problems are annoying for everyone, but they represent higher risk for vocalists. If general wellness habits aren't enough to resolve them, then medical or surgical help may be worth the trouble.

All things share the same breath—the beast, the tree, the man, they all share the same breath.
—Chief Seattle

6

Food

The best doctors in the world are Doctor Diet,
Doctor Quiet, and Doctor Merryman.
—Jonathan Swift

Our lives are not in the lap of the gods,
but in the lap of our cooks.
—Lin Yutang

I prithee go and get me some repast;
I care not what, so it be wholesome food.
—From *The Taming of the Shrew*, by William Shakespeare

You Don't Talk Where You Swallow

The most important job that the voice box (*larynx*) performs in the body is to keep food and liquid out of the lungs. Look back at Fig. 1 in chapter 2, "How the Voice Works": your mouth and throat lead into the pathways for both breathing and swallowing.

At the larynx, those passages divide and remain separate. Your voice box, by its position and action, serves as the switching station between these pathways. This is central to its biological job of protecting the airway.

Most of the time, your airway is open and your esophagus (the tube from your throat to your stomach) is closed. At the moment of swallowing, the voice box closes the airway completely so that what you swallow doesn't "go down the wrong way."

Put simply, under normal circumstances, nothing that you eat or drink directly touches the vocal folds. If something enters your airway by mistake, your body coughs it out to prevent choking and to keep your lungs clean.

Nevertheless, the pathways for eating and for breathing or voicing are so close together that it is easy to believe or imagine that drinking or eating something can make your voice better. This is one instance where common sense is wrong! If hot tea, honey, or anything else seems to feel good in the throat, that nice sensation is usually about an inch away from the vocal cords—a big distance in that part of the body.

Beverages, medicines, and common home remedies taken by mouth may contain helpful ingredients, but none of these substances directly "wets" or "lubricates" the vocal cords. Their benefits are indirect, as the chemicals are processed through digestion.

So although it's fine to eat things that feel good—steamy soup in cold weather or iced sherbet when your throat is hot and dry—the more important principle is to choose foods based on overall health rather on than what might feel good for an instant on your throat. As discussed in chapter 5, "Air," your voice is kept more directly comfortable by how you use it and by what's in the air.

Stamina, Protection, and Space

When choosing a way of eating that enhances your vocal health, there are three main principles to follow: maximize general wellness and stamina, guard against acid reflux irritation of the vocal cords, and keep the digestive system comfortable rather than overstuffed. The oft-stated lore that vocalists should avoid dairy products also deserves some attention, although this is another instance where the most accurate research information may not match other things you've been told.

A healthy voice requires a strong body with generally good muscle tone and endurance. So plan to eat a balance of protein, fruits and vegetables, whole grains and beans, and moderate amounts of healthy fats and oils.

There are plenty of books and beliefs about the best way to select food. In my experience, individual bodies vary. Some people feel energized by protein rather than carbohydrate fuel, while others feel weighed down by meat and prefer lighter fare. Pay attention to how you feel and experiment until you find a food regimen that suits your own body, schedule, and budget. Consult with a dietician or nutritionist for individualized help.

Your Throat on Acid

As shown in Fig. 1, chapter 2, "How Your Voice Works," the larynx is very close to the esophagus. In fact, only a few layers of tissue separate them. If a small amount of stomach acid sneaks back up the esophagus (a process called *reflux*) and gets all the way up to the throat, it is likely to "land" at the back area of the vocal cords. This condition—called *laryngo-pharyngeal reflux* (LPR)—is not good for your voice!

The breathing and swallowing tubes have different jobs, so they are lined with different kinds of cells. The inside of the digestive system has special buffers against the strong acids and other materials that do the work of digestion. The inside of the larynx and lower airway don't have this protection.

Acid material refluxing from the stomach and falling onto the vocal folds will irritate or burn them. One such episode can have effects on the voice that last for days, and repeated episodes over time can cause vocal changes and discomfort that are generally called *reflux laryngitis*.

This condition is diagnosed by a laryngologist based on your symptoms, the appearance of your vocal folds on a visual exam, and whether certain medications make things better. Some patients with reflux irritation of the voice (LPR) report stomach discomfort, burning sensations, acidic taste in the mouth, and so on, but most do not.

Thus acid-related vocal inflammation often occurs without any familiar symptoms of heartburn. (This is yet another area in which your common sense and your internal sensations can be plain wrong. Remember that parts of these body functions are designed to be unconscious, so you just can't feel everything accurately.)

The digestive and respiratory systems are close enough together in the laryngeal region to influence each other, even though their functions are different. With LPR, the source of the problem is in the digestive system, but the symptoms are experienced in the voice and upper throat.

Ironically, singers and vigorous talkers are believed to be at higher risk for reflux because of the active pressure changes inside the body from deeper breathing, singing, and forceful speech. Acid reflux is also more common in women than men, in people over age 35, in those who are overweight, and during periods of high emotional stress.

Common complaints with LPR include a gradual roughening of the voice (hoarseness) that seems independent of overuse or any lingering cold, and the sensation of a thickening or lump in the throat. Patients say, "There's just something in there." I see and hear a lot of throat clearing from these patients, but when I ask if it really helps, they admit it doesn't. You can't cough out a condition of being swollen or irritated!

The voice can sound low pitched and crackly, and it can get tired more easily, as the condition of laryngeal reflux becomes more serious or long-standing and untreated. Singers with LPR may find that the midrange is harder to control, in contrast with other vocal problems that tend to hurt the upper range first. Chronic cough and other breathing problems can also develop.

But not everyone has the same symptoms, and it is time to repeat that you cannot diagnose your own voice problems by sound or feel. These descriptions of possible symptoms or complaints are offered so that, if you experience these things, you pay attention to them and can describe them to your doctor.

Doctors generally agree on the examination signs that are likely to indicate LPR, but some of these signs are the same as allergic inflammation, so it can get tricky. If antireflux medications are effective in resolving your throat symptoms, the diagnosis is confirmed.

A few doctors disagree with the whole concept, or fear that the condition is now overdiagnosed. Gastro-intestinal (GI) specialists remain skeptical in many cases, because they are not trained to observe the larynx. This is more good reason to be examined by an MD who is a real voice specialist and has experience sorting out such problems.

If laryngeal reflux is left untreated, more serious vocal problems can develop over time, such as a benign but painful sore on one or both vocal cords (*granuloma*). In the most extreme cases, uncontrolled acid reflux can contribute to laryngeal cancer.

Most of the time, laryngeal reflux is mild and easily managed, usually with a combination of medication, diet, and lifestyle changes. If you are given this diagnosis, your doctor or speech pathologist will provide you with individualized information.

The Antireflux Regimen

He who takes medicine and neglects his diet
wastes the skill of his doctors.
—Chinese proverb

If you've been diagnosed with acid-reflux problems, you may be advised to manage it with diet alone or with one or more medications. Note that this is still a topic of ongoing research; experts disagree, and as usual, the Internet will offer you multiple, conflicting points of view. Do the best you can within your own lifestyle and according to your vocal demands, and find out over time what works for you.

Keep in mind, though, that reflux irritations don't heal overnight. You may have to modify your diet or follow a medication routine for four to eight weeks before you and your doctor know if it's even beginning to be helpful. If you need a few days to adjust to the diagnosis and new routine, stay diligent and patient as the symptoms start to resolve.

Here are some current dietary guidelines for reflux management:

- Limit or eliminate alcoholic beverages, coffee, citrus and tomato foods and juices, and extremely fatty or spicy foods. (The latest information on coffee is that it may not cause reflux, but it worsens reflux problems that already exist. Decaffeinated coffee and tea appear to be less of a problem; we don't know for sure.)

- Soda and other sparkling beverages can increase pressure in the stomach and make reflux episodes more likely. Decrease these too, especially at night and before a performance.

- Don't eat late at night; if you have an evening snack, make it small and easily digestible, and sit up for a while after you eat, before going to bed. Depending on the severity of your problem, your doctor may recommend that you wait two to four hours after you eat before going to sleep.

People with reflux problems are sometimes advised to elevate the head of the bed, so that during the night, gravity helps keep stomach juices where they belong. This appears to be less relevant for the specific type of reflux that afflicts the vocal cords. But depending on the severity of your symptoms and your doctor's clinical opinion, it may be recommended.

If you decide to angle your bed, it's important to use a wedge-shaped pillow or blocks under the head of your bed. Propping up just your head on extra pillows tends to squeeze the midsection of the body, which makes reflux worse rather than better.

The initial stage of treatment may last for six months. The more careful you are, the more sure you and your doctor can be about what's working. This can feel like quite a long, frustrating process, but many voice patients ultimately feel a huge benefit in both sound and sensation. Professional speakers, vocal artists, and outgoing folks who just love to use their voices will especially find the challenge to be worthwhile.

If giving up favorite foods and drinks feels as though it would be impossible for you to do, be honest with yourself and just do the absolute best you can. Make gradual but steady changes, getting closer and closer to your doctor's recommendation. Review the guidelines frequently to see what's working and how you can further improve your daily habits. "I screwed up again" is a very different motivator than the calm, compassionate self-care that truly helps your voice.

Some holistic-health specialists deny the problem of acid reflux or warn of horrible side effects from the most common antireflux medications. The latest research—as of this writing—indicates that long-term use of some reflux medications does have side effects, but "long-term" here means "many years." But if there is no benefit from —three to six months of treatment, along with diligent lifestyle changes and the most advanced antireflux medications, the problem is probably not reflux, and MDs will reconsider the prescription.

Emotional stress may or may not cause stomach problems, but it certainly keeps your body from recovering and repairing from acid and other irritants. Smoking has also been proven to increase the risk of acid reflux; this is one more good reason to quit.

Unstuffing

Your voice works best when your digestive system is comfortable and not too full. In the midsection of the body, digestion and breathing compete for space. Big meals take up space below your diaphragm, making it harder for the breathing muscles to work. Extra gas from carbonated drinks or beer can have the same effect.

You also don't want to be too empty or hungry before a performance or an important speech because this can make you mentally spacey or physically weak. Small meals and snacks spaced throughout the day are commonly recommended by nutritionists to keep your energy steady. This approach will also help you achieve consistent breath support.

Those who perform at night are often tempted to eat a large meal after the show. This refueling can feel like a psychological reward as well as a time of social bonding after hours of hard teamwork. But a heavy meal, especially with alcoholic drinks, increases the risk of acid reflux overnight and can disrupt the sleep you need just as much.

Try having a smaller snack after the show (soup, fruit, yogurt, cereal) with minimal alcohol. Finish unwinding with a shower (steam treatment) and meditative breathing exercises. Plan on a bigger breakfast the next morning (or light breakfast and substantial lunch) as your main daily fuel.

Got Milk Worries?

Many voice students are told to avoid milk, cheese, and other dairy products. Usually, the explanation is that milk in some way increases mucous (phlegm) or makes it thicker.

You may be surprised to learn that according to the latest research, the only people whose phlegm changes in the presence of dairy products are those who expect and believe in this relationship! Yet this belief is so deep in vocal lore that giving up dairy can become a signal of someone taking his or her voice seriously.

There are lots of theories about the effect of milk enzymes in the mouth or digestive tract, and all have been disproven by scientific research in biochemistry. I've learned this since the earlier version of this book, and I too was surprised. The research is pretty clear, though, no matter that it goes against a strong rule in the subculture of voice.

So what's a diligent vocalist to do? If you're not sure about how dairy products affect your voice but have an open mind, the best advice is to experiment. Avoid all dairy products for four to six hours before a few practice sessions and performances, without changing

One Physician's Formula for Healthy Eating

Ray Sahelian, MD, runs a thoughtful website on natural healing called Advance Physician Formulas, at www.physicianformulas.com. In the spring of 2011, a letter was published in his newsletter from a reader who proclaimed that dairy products are harmful for everyone and that Sahelian's website should say so. Dr. Sahelian's responded with the following:

"One can find something wrong with just about almost every food group. People worry about fish due to contamination and high levels of mercury. Many people think soy is a poison. Our meats and chickens could have hormones. Vegetables and fruits could have pesticides and at times carry germs that cause deadly infections. Some people think we should not eat grains since these have been introduced to the human diet for only a few thousand years and the body has not adapted to them. Well.

anything else in your normal routine. If you find that your voice works significantly better in a dairy-free zone, you can choose to make this change part of your normal healthy-voice plan, being sure to replace milk with other sources of protein and calcium.

You have the right to your own food preferences, based on taste, culture, family habit, friends, and life circumstances. I wouldn't instruct any vocal performer that they should drink milk.

If your voice seems to work the same regardless of dairy ingredients, don't let your self-knowledge or confidence be shaken by someone else's beliefs. If, on the

"I don't think it is worthwhile to go through life constantly worrying about all the possible dangers lurking in our foods (unless a person is clearly allergic to certain food components). I know people who avoid one or two major food groups such as dairy or grains, but then they end up consuming more sweets and sugars that make their health even worse. For practical purposes I tell my patients to select as much organic foods as possible, to consume a wide variety of foods in balanced proportions, and not to get too obsessed about this issue."

other hand, your identity as a performer or as a health-conscious person includes avoiding dairy products, that remains your choice.

My view is very much like Dr. Sahelian's. I feel sad when singing students seem to have heard stronger lectures about avoiding milk than about trusting their own bodies and health signals. Common sense puts dairy foods in context, as one element among many that might influence your vocal health and performance. So please work as hard on stress management, self-respect, and vocal technique as you do on avoiding dairy products or controlling other elements of your diet.

What's This About Nuts?

A final food note: Some music or choral teachers instruct singers to avoid eating nuts, especially before a performance. To the best of my knowledge, this is not based on nutrition or chemistry; nuts are currently considered a good source of protein and "healthy" oils.

However, unless you floss and brush your teeth thoroughly between eating nuts and singing, small hard particles can remain in the mouth and fly into the larynx on a vigorous inhalation. The subsequent coughing fit is both unpleasant and disruptive to a concert. Nuts are otherwise a handy snack, so just be careful!

Chapter 6 Summary

- To develop an optimal eating plan for voice care, start by understanding your individual allergies, preferences, budget, and beliefs about food.

- Follow general nutrition guidelines so that you have the physical stamina your voice needs and a balance of nutrients.

- Take reasonable precautions against acid reflux, such as not going to sleep after a large meal, to prevent future problems. If you are already struggling with your voice and are given this diagnosis, talk honestly with your doctor about specific antireflux recommendations.

- Stay open-minded about the "dairy dilemma." Remember how much "information" about voice care comes from centuries before there was any science. Make choices that keep you confident as well as healthy.

- Food is important, but it's only one ingredient in the voice-care recipe.

7

Drink

Water is the driving force of all nature.
—Leonardo da Vinci

I'm an instant star. Just add water and stir.
—David Bowie

No Substitute

Most serious talkers and singers have already heard that it's important to drink a lot of water. This water does not directly "wet" the vocal folds. Swallowing water sends it down the other tube, the esophagus, into your stomach.

Drinking plenty of water does make sure that the cells inside the voice box are nourished and resilient. If the body as a whole is dehydrated, the vocal folds get tired faster, and they recover more slowly from heavy use.

Recommendations on the right amount of water intake range

from two quarts or two liters per day to "whatever it takes to pee pale." The latest guideline I've heard of is to divide your weight in pounds by 2 and drink that number of ounces (see the sidebar below). Sipping your water throughout the day and evening is much more beneficial than trying to drink a lot all at once.

People have different internal sensations of thirst, or desire for water. If your voice is working well, you may already get enough for your own system. If you notice signs of vocal fatigue and you're not in the habit of staying hydrated, increasing the amount of water you drink is a simple first step to try.

As always, use common sense. If you have heart or kidney problems, or other concerns about fluid intake, talk to your doctor before making drastic changes.

Suggested Daily Fluid Guidelines

Hydration in ounces per day per pound of body weight

If you weigh,

    100 lbs: aim to drink 50 oz, about 3 pints

    125 lbs: aim to drink 62 oz, about 2 quarts

    150 lbs: aim to drink 75 oz, about 5 pints

    200 lbs: aim to drink 100 oz, about 3 quarts

Hydration in liters per day per kg of body weight

If you weigh,

    45 kg: aim to drink about 1.5 liters

    60 kg: aim to drink about 2.0 liters

    80 kg: aim to drink about 2.5 liters

    100 kg: aim to drink about 3.0 liters

Ice-cold drinks used to be forbidden to serious vocalists. However, research has shown that it doesn't matter whether you drink cold, hot, warm, or lukewarm beverages during rehearsal and performance.

Drink whatever temperature you like, what feels best on a particular day. The main thing is to get plenty of fluids on a regular basis.

Coffee and Other Culprits

The beverages to avoid are those that contain alcohol or caffeine, especially coffee. These chemicals draw water out of the body, so they do not count toward your daily water "ration." Eliminate them if you can, or cut back gradually, and drink enough water to compensate.

As explained in chapter 6, "Food," coffee increases the severity of acid reflux. Tea and decaffeinated coffee appear to be safer. Coffee and other caffeinated beverages also disrupt sleep, and they can increase anxiety and stage-fright-related symptoms. Many of my patients say they need caffeine boosts because they don't sleep well—but perhaps they are not sleeping well because of drinking so much coffee!

I worked with a businessman who complained of vocal fatigue, and he was in the habit of drinking coffee throughout the day. He drank very little water.

When he got into the habit of keeping water at his desk, he was surprised at how refreshing it could be. He found that his voice did not tire out as easily when he sipped water throughout the day and drank less coffee. He slept better, and within a month his overall energy improved so that he felt less need for a caffeine boost, even in the late afternoon.

The thirsty earth soaks up the rain,
And drinks, and gapes for drink again;
The plants suck in the earth, and are
With constant drinking fresh and fair.
—Abraham Cowley

Liquid Courage (Not)

Alcoholic beverages are generally discouraged for the serious voice user. The combined risks of dehydration, acid reflux, and uninhibited voice overuse are rarely worth it. When friends around you are drinking, you can switch to water or soda and they probably won't notice.

An occasional cocktail, beer, or glass of wine may not be a problem if your voice is otherwise working well. Just be sure that you're getting enough fluid in other forms, and that you're not relying on alcohol to medicate stage fright; there are better ways to relax that don't carry the risks of throat problems or chemical addiction. More on this topic in chapter 22, "Tobacco, Alcohol, and Marijuana."

Soda and Sport Drinks

Carbonated sodas are discouraged by some voice experts because the extra fullness in the stomach competes with more basic needs for breathing and digestion. Drinking soda before a rehearsal or performance can impair good breath technique, not to mention increasing the risks of belching in the middle of a phrase.

As an alternative to carbonated soft drinks, performing artists (and others pressured to work long hours with inadequate rest) increasingly favor specially marketed sport, "energy," or herbal beverages. These formulas are typically based on sugar and caffeine, sometimes in an herbal form, such as guarana, plus herbs or vitamins that promise to increase "pep." But this "energy" is not free—it is borrowed from the future. Such drinks can leave you too wired to sleep well, increasing your fatigue for the next day or even week.

The formulas advertised for weight loss may be lower in sugar than the rest, but high in potassium, a diuretic. Or they may be even higher in caffeine or herbal stimulants. Some ingredients have negative side effects on mood or just may not agree with your individual chemistry. Know what you are putting into your body, and why! If a doctor or other voice professional asks you about how much coffee you drink, be sure to include all sodas and energy drinks in your response.

If these beverages have been in your lifestyle for a long time when you decide to cut back, it may be better to ease off in stages rather than stopping suddenly. For instance, dilute them half and half with water for a couple of weeks, or switch to plain water after lunch. As always, know yourself and what works for you.

The simplest sports drinks are designed to replace sugar and electrolytes (minerals) lost during hard exercise. Unless you also dance for hours every day or exercise heavily, these drinks are not typically necessary for singers or talkers.

The newest "vitamin waters" have no evidence of being harmful. They're just expensive and unnecessary. Fresh juicy fruits and vegetables (melon, cucumber, apples, pears, jicama, and so on) can help keep your mouth moist and your body generally hydrated; they also contain fiber (protective against reflux) and micronutrients that are not found in the vitamin drinks.

Thousands have lived without love, not one without water.

—W. H. Auden

Chapter 7 Summary

- Sip water steadily throughout the day to keep your vocal tissues hydrated.

- Cold, hot, warm, and even ice-cold beverages are all okay. Use whatever temperature you like the best.

- Beverages with caffeine or alcohol don't count toward your daily fluid intake needs.

- Peppy sports drinks loaded with caffeine, herbs, and vitamins are unnecessary and expensive.

- Fresh, watery fruits and vegetables can help you stay hydrated as well as nourished.

8

Voice Rest

Choose silence of all virtues, for by it you hear other
men's imperfections, and conceal your own.
—George Bernard Shaw

When you talk or sing, the surfaces of your vocal cords vibrate
against each other 100 to 1,000 times per second. As described in chapter 1, "Consciousness and Contradictions,"
the active support muscles switch on and off multiple times per
second to position the vocal cords and shape the various sounds of
speech.

The vocal mechanism is built to handle these jobs, just not all the
time, with no chance to recover. Even the most talented, best-trained
voices need rest as part of general preventative care. Your voice will
stay healthier when allowed opportunities to rest, recover, rehydrate,
and relax.

This can simply mean taking short breaks throughout the day, especially if your job requires constant talking (such as teaching, sales,
broadcasting, and customer service). If you've been lecturing or singing for an hour, don't use up your entire rest break talking, even if
people really want your attention. Your voice needs attention, too.

When you have a big vocal demand coming up, build in rest periods before and after. If you have extremely heavy vocal demands (for example, vocal performances every night with all-day rehearsals, business meetings, or a speech-heavy daytime job), try to set aside one full day per week for silent rest.

After all, star athletes have built-in rest days, or they play in rotation. If you are a vocal athlete, your throat needs the same care.

What about resting the voice when there's a problem, such as vocal nodules? Medical opinion on this has changed over the years; you can search online and find every possible recommendation.

In the early days of voice care, when there was a problem with the voice, doctors would often prescribe complete silence for a month or more. That might have worked for people with servants and no children, but it is no longer considered realistic or necessary in most cases. Extended silence can even lead to a fear that the voice will "break" when speech resumes.

Vocal rest recommendations are now more individualized. The physiological benefits of voice rest are balanced with its psychological, interpersonal, and vocational costs.

For diagnosed problems related to overuse, vocal rest is usually combined with rehabilitation (retraining). Your own doctor and speech therapist will determine your best plan.

This is ideally a process of negotiation and problem solving, not just being given a list of rules by someone in a white coat! For instance, if heavy use is built into your job, the speech therapist can help you sort through each speech situation by its vocal risks and demands, prioritizing so you use your "vocal allowance" on the most important tasks.

This might mean that you eliminate the most intense vocal demands (yelling, singing, lecturing without a microphone), cut all phone calls in half, and schedule several short breaks for silent rest. Another guideline for those with simple voice injuries is to "talk half as much and half as loud."

Sometimes, the "silence treatment" is non-negotiable. For instance, after vocal surgery your doctor may prescribe a week or two of strict voice rest so that the vibratory edges of the vocal folds can heal properly. Vocal-fold hemorrhages and some kinds of burns (thermal trauma) also typically need a period of absolute rest. It's important to follow such instructions to avoid serious complications or permanent vocal damage.

Even before you see a doctor, giving yourself complete vocal rest for a day or two may be helpful if you've had an unexpected vocal strain. See chapter 11, "First Aid for Hoarseness," for more on this.

Rest Strategies

Even when you understand your doctor's and therapist's recommendations, reducing the amount that you talk or sing can be difficult, given the demands of jobs, school, and family. Especially now that cell phones go with us everywhere, it can be disorienting to stop talking (see chapter 18, "Telephones and Other Electronics"). The central role the voice plays in our lives as social creatures is never so clear as when it's taken away.

Isolation from your closest relationships or fears about not fulfilling job obligations can interfere with the subtler levels of healing. This is one reason that medical recommendations about extended voice rest have shifted. Partial, strategic rest helps you value your voice without damaging your most important relationships or developing an irrational fear of talking.

Nevertheless, friends and family may need to have multiple reminders about what you are doing. Reassure them that you still care for them, but that you need to stay connected without "using up" your voice. Similarly, employers may need to know that the situation is temporary and that you're willing to take on other responsibilities with less vocal demand.

Texting and email alternatives have made vocal rest much easier than in past decades. But they don't make up for simply talking, especially for older relatives or those without access to the latest technology.

As one patient told me, "My friends are cool about this vocal rest thing. They understand and even remind me to be quiet when I get into that husky spot. But when I make my weekly phone call to my mom and tell her I can only talk for five minutes, she doesn't really get it. She says she loves me and needs to hear my voice."

Although not a perfect solution, it may help to email or send postcards to such people more often than usual. Ask those close to you who do understand to give extra attention to the people who feel deprived by your silence.

Do your best to cultivate patience, and learn from the experience of extended vocal rest so that you won't need to go through it again. The more diligent you are with voice rest when it's recommended, the faster you'll heal and return to your network of spoken connections.

In ancient times, purposeful solitude was both palliative and preventive . . . a way of listening to the inner self to solicit advice and guidance otherwise impossible to hear in the din of daily life.

—Clarissa Pinkola Estés

I have often regretted my speech, never my silence.

—Publilius Syrus

Singers, actors, and professional speakers taking vocal rest can still rehearse mentally, as athletes do. Go through a warm-up routine or performance in your imagination. If you concentrate fully, a mental performance builds the same brain pathways as a "real" one. Quiet days are also a good time to write or edit material, to study texts or music that you need to memorize, or to work on your press kit.

Another good use of vocal rest time, especially if your voice is struggling a bit, is to mentally scan your body for injuries, illnesses, or weaknesses that might have snuck up on you, weakening your voice or compromising technique. Do the same for emotional or relationship stress factors that may feel lodged in your body.

The voice can be a sensitive indicator of overall wellness or physiological stress, and in these cases its distress sounds are a call for help from the rest of your body-mind. Mentally thank your voice for bringing these issues to your attention, and make plans to deal with them as soon as you can.

Once my patients decide to give their voices more rest, many of them are amazed and pleased that their communication actually improves. They learn how to make careful choices about what's important to say and when listening is enough.

They become more conscious of when they talk to fill time or to ease boredom or anxiety, rather than to convey information or develop an important relationship. They also start to value the silent time for reflection and relaxation.

Sleep

Sleep is the body's chance to rebuild cells and organs, replace worn-out tissues, and restore both mental and metabolic equilibrium. Your voice benefits from all of this. World-class tenor and conductor Placido Domingo was once asked whether he had a secret way to keep his voice in top form. He answered, "Before a performance, I make sure to sleep 11 hours!"

You may not need that much, but sleeping for seven or eight hours regularly may be an important piece of your voice-care plan. The dietary guidelines that appear booking chapter 6, "Food"—minimal caffeine and alcohol, no big meals before bed—will help you get good-quality sleep.

Chapter 8 Summary

- Routinely rest your voice for short periods throughout the day—for instance, five minutes per hour. This relaxes the muscles in your throat and gives the vibrating edges a chance to rebuild.

- Build longer rest breaks into the schedule of vocal rehearsals, performances, or other vocally demanding work.

- When voice trouble strikes, negotiate with family, friends, and coworkers about your needs for silent rest and how else you can communicate.

- If a doctor prescribes absolute vocal rest for a specific injury, follow the rules to avoid more serious or prolonged problems.

- Use vocal rest for mental rehearsal and other career-supporting tasks, as well as for silent reflection and self-discovery.

- Nourish the cells of your voice box most deeply with adequate sleep.

A field that has rested gives a bountiful crop.

—Ovid

9

Exercise

Talking is a physiologically demanding activity, with major effects on the cardiovascular system. It increases blood pressure, heart rate, and arrhythmia . . . even [when] about nonstressful subjects.

—Anne Karpf

Those who think they have not time for bodily exercise will sooner or later have to find time for illness.

—Edward Stanley

As I emphasize throughout this book, vocal health reflects the overall health of the body. Physical exercise gives us vitality, bodily resilience, and mental benefits that are perhaps more important for vocalists than for the average person.

For vocalists, some fitness activities are more directly useful than others. Other types of exercise put the vocal cords at risk. Few fitness instructors are trained in these areas, so you need to bring your own vocal wisdom to the gym, sports field, or dance or yoga studio.

Many voice students I know, like other citizens of our fast-paced modern world, find it hard to get the amount of regular exercise recommended by health experts, even if they may personally enjoy it. If it's hard for you to find time for fitness, it's that much more important to use your time well in activities that best support your vocal health.

Good for You

The most basic fitness contribution to the voice is cardio-vascular endurance or general stamina. Whether you're an actor or opera singer expected to clamber around fantastical sets created by hip designers, a rocker maneuvering stage equipment and effects while dancing, or an attorney or business speaker seeking to command a room through physical as well as vocal presence, you'll be served well by any activities that offer a balance of cardio fitness, flexibility and agility, and muscle toning. In fact, enthusiastic opera singers helped to popularize jogging a decade before Jane Fonda's workout videos made aerobics a household word.

If you think that it's hard to find time for exercise, here's a story that may help motivate you. Rock singer Bret Michaels made headlines in 2010 for a series of medical emergencies, including surgeries to his abdomen, brain, and heart. Yet by April 2011, he was back on tour, and he explained to US Weekly magazine that living out of a tour bus didn't stop him from the exercise his body needed. "I get out at every truck stop in America and throw footballs or baseballs or ride my bike. That's how I stay healthy," he says.

Another important benefit of physical activity is to support effective management of the vocal breath by developing a balance of flexibility and power in the rib cage, waist, and abdomen (more on this below). Fitness activities can also enhance your sense of body rhythm, postural balance, and awareness of subtle energy flows, all of which benefit the voice.

On the other hand, it's important for people who depend on their voices to recognize where fitness activities and vocal development can conflict. Avoiding neck constriction or harsh, explosive vocalizing during exercise are especially important precautions to take. More-subtle concerns are outer vs. inner mental focus, breath rhythm, and how much the voice itself is valued.

Compare and Contrast

Traditional sports, such as swimming, tennis, soccer, and basketball, as well as dance and aerobics classes, certainly build stamina and strong, efficient breathing—all good for voice, too. Notice, though, that during this kind of sport or dance activity, most of your mental focus is external—what's happening around you. You may attend to the position of your arms and legs when learning new skills, but you use those skills toward an external goal.

By contrast, vocal activity happens at the center of the body and is largely out of sight. The brain sends and receives vocal messages through parts of the nervous system that are partly conscious and partly unconscious and visceral.

So if developing and protecting your voice are your primary goals, find occasional moments during exercise to turn your mind inward. For instance, observe whether you feel more connected to your lower body or upper body, whether your eye gaze is in close-up or faraway mode, or whether your breathing is silent or audible. The details of what you monitor aren't as important as the process of enhancing awareness of your inner body while engaging in a vigorous activity.

Especially practice this mindful, nonjudgmental thought process while cooling down and transitioning from vigorous exercise to other activities. Learning to balance your inner and outer attention while the body is busy and metabolically active will serve your voice in profound ways.

After every workout, take time to stretch your neck, back, shoulders, chest, and the muscles around your rib cage. Stretch your abdominal muscles and learn how to relax as well as tighten them; a strong voice needs both.

Breathing, Again

Another fundamental difference between voice training and most fitness activities lies in breath rhythm. During most physical exercise, we use a relatively simple breath rhythm; inhalation and exhalation are roughly equal in length.

When talking or singing, however, the breath rhythm is always unequal: the inhalation is swift and the exhalation slow. So while many activities may strengthen your breathing muscles, only a few, such as swimming, reinforce the specific breath control needed for voice. Just being aware of the difference—like sensing the difference between outer and inner attention—can be useful.

You can also modify some cardio activities, practicing intervals of "voice breath." For instance, instead of matching to the same number of steps when breathing in and breathing out, try inhaling quickly and exhaling over a longer number of steps. This won't work if you're exercising at peak intensity; your body's demand for oxygen and ventilation will override any other breath adjustments.

Try it during lower-intensity activities or intervals, and you'll feel muscles in the waist and rib-cage area fighting hard to keep your lungs fuller, longer. Or simply try singing, talking, or chanting as you exercise, and the breath rhythm will adjust by itself.

I admit that this will slow down the aerobics; for top cardiovascular conditioning, the experts warn against trying to converse while you're working out! Consider it a vocal-needs variation that helps you balance physical fitness with vocal fitness and sharpen your awareness of both.

I taught this uneven-breath technique to a sportscaster I coached years ago, who loved the microphone and the gym equally. He was thrilled at being able to develop both areas of strength at the same time.

Specific athletic activities, such as diving, use breathing techniques for safety and coordination, especially at the elite level. While the details may not match what's best for your voice, the process of coordinating breath with other physical actions will serve your voice. Again, just stay aware of the differences in use so you can switch mental gears as you change activities.

Finally, learn to keep your breath silent even during a hard workout. The sound of turbulence in your throat means that your airway is not completely open, and your vocal cords may get roughed up or unnecessarily dry from the air.

It is exercise alone that supports the spirits,
and keeps the mind in vigor.
—Marcus Tullius Cicero

Play Hard, Take Care

The last significant difference between voice care and general exercise principles is that in sports or gym workouts, voice use supports the other activities and may even be sacrificed for them. Cheering, coaching, venting emotion, or punctuating key moments—vocal expression in the fitness world is typically loud, explosive, and expected to be automatic. Vocal overuse and hoarseness may be expected, if not rewarded, as signs of commitment, team spirit, selflessness, and other values.

If "playing while hurt" is a conscious sacrifice sometimes demanded of athletes and dancers, "playing while hoarse" isn't even noticed. Even worse, the internal nature of voice and the historical lack of information about it can frame concern about vocal health as weak, selfish, and nonmacho.

People committed to a variety of activities, vocal and not—or who just need something left vocally for work or family communication after a game—do not typically get much understanding or support. All the more reason for you to thoroughly understand self-care principles and carefully develop your own strategies.

I worked with a teenage girl whose twin ambitions were musical theater and volleyball. During practice as well as tournaments, her volleyball coach demanded that players not currently on the court cheer and scream for their teammates. Those who didn't yell loudly enough were kept on the bench and not given a turn to play.

Naturally, her singing voice suffered. Only when several families with the same dilemma got together to talk to the coach did he grudgingly allow the girls to prove their team loyalty in nonvocal ways.

Cheerleaders and athletes expected to shout during the game and not allowed such compromises should warm up their voices as well as their bodies. Limit how much you talk over noise at postgame parties, and steam your throat as often as you ice your muscle aches.

Those who coach athletics, especially outdoors, are at high risk for vocal strain and overuse injuries. As much as possible, save your voice for meaningful communication rather than long-distance signaling. Use a whistle to get players' attention and a megaphone or portable microphone and speaker to project and protect your voice.

Whatever your favorite sport or fitness activity, protect your voice. Don't shout over loud music just because a fitness teacher wants you to. If you dance and sing at the same time, work with an experienced coach to master the special breathing techniques that serve both your voice and your needs as a dancer.

Mind and Body Together

The best forms of physical exercise for vocalists are those that integrate the body, mind, and breath, helping to harmonize conscious and unconscious functions. When I studied acting at CalArts, we were required to take tai chi every year, and it was my favorite preparation for voice class. Qigong and, of course, yoga, are similarly powerful.

If available in your community, I encourage you to explore these and similar approaches to body awareness and conditioning in addition to your favorite method of more vigorous cardio fitness. Practiced regularly, they can support vocal training in profound and subtle ways.

Question from an Online Forum: Neck Stiffness from Exercise

I do a lot of physical training, and while I try, I can't always keep my neck relaxed. I don't talk, grunt, or close my throat, and yet my voice sometimes feels tight and restricted even after my abdomen has recovered. Is there anything else I can do to stop from putting stress on my voice while I work out?

My Suggestions

- **Find exercises that specifically relax your throat** (tongue stretching, yawn, slow or silent breath, throat massage) and use them before and after your workout and during rest breaks.
- **Move your head around.** Roll it back and forth on the bench, or in little circles, during the strength-training moves. This will isolate your neck from the rest of the effort. Try the same thing with easy vocal warm-ups. If you can't do an exercise while you move your head and make comfortable sound, reduce the weight. Harder on the ego, better on the voice.
- **Focus on muscle relationships and balance between the neck and the jaw.** Sometimes, the jaw acts as an extra stabilizer for the upper body, clenching during heavy workouts, and this can add tension to the voice and breath. To unlearn this habit you may need to reduce the intensity of your workout, and give up that teeth-gritting look of aggression. But your athletic form will actually become more precise, and your throat will benefit.
- **If you still notice problems, ask your doctor for a physical-therapy referral.** A few sessions of muscle treatment and troubleshooting your routine could help a lot, and a good physical therapist knows details that your gym buddies won't.

Fitness Activities

Abdominal Strengthening

Good for voice: Posture, appearance, breath awareness; keeps back healthy and strong.

Cautions and comments: Don't hold your breath during these (or any other) exercises. Breathe as silently as possible. Learn to isolate the lowest or deepest muscle layer ("transverse abdominal") from the long ("rectus") and oblique muscles. The transverse is most important to posture and breath control, but it becomes weak if ignored in favor of a "six-pack" or tiny waist. You should be able to breathe fully around or behind your "core." After the workout, stretch and relax the abdominal area as deeply as you worked it.

Aerobic Conditioning or "Cardio" (for example, running, bicycling, stairs, elliptical machines, jump-rope)

Good for voice: Heart-lung fitness; strengthens breathing muscles; builds stamina for vocal performance.

Cautions and comments: Keep throat wide open (silent) when you inhale. High-intensity exercise may engage vigorous breathing high in the chest; this type of expansion is not so good for voice, so be conscious of the difference. In biking and spinning, oblique abdominals may become overtrained and the back of the neck tight. As described above, during any aerobic workout, try short intervals of asymmetrical breathing (in=fast/out=slow) to support the rhythm and control needed for voice.

Dance

Good for voice: Cardio conditioning, posture, flexibility, appearance; trains the body to respond to music.

Cautions and comments: Keep throat wide open (silent) when you inhale. Don't talk, yell, or teach over loud music without a microphone. Occasionally relax or soften abdomen to keep space available for vocal support.

Martial Arts

Good for voice: Aerobic fitness, flexibility, mind-body connection, subtle energy circulation, "soft belly" with low center of gravity.

Cautions and comments: Keep throat wide open (silent) when you inhale. Teacher may request shouts and grunts; make comfortable sounds but don't push too much. Learning to keep your throat and jaw relaxed can be part of the energy awareness of your practice.

Swimming

Good for voice: Typically uses "in-fast/out-slow" breath rhythm, very similar to vocal performance; builds endurance like other aerobics, with good shoulder and rib cage flexibility; possibly the best exercise activity for voice professionals.

Cautions and comments: Keep neck relaxed. Chlorine in water is irritating to some people, leading to a sore-throat feeling. Discuss this with your doctor. If the swim facility has a steam room, use it!

Strength Training (calisthenics, weights)

Good for voice: Overall fitness, joint support, injury recovery, appearance.

Cautions and comments: Don't hold your breath, even if that means lifting less weight. Don't exhale on exertion;

start exhaling before the push. Avoid any grunts or audible expulsions of breath. Stay conscious of neck muscles while working other body areas; keep neck and jaw relaxed at all times. After strengthening, spend generous time stretching for maximum freedom and ease of movement.

Tai Chi, Qigong

Good for voice: Low-impact aerobic fitness, flexibility, mind-body connection, subtle-energy circulation, "soft-belly" with low center of gravity.

Cautions and comments: Some specialized qigong healing techniques involve tightening the throat muscles to hold breath and "compress" the air in the body. If you practice this, be sure to relax the throat fully afterward. Otherwise, these practices are among the best forms of fitness exercise for vocalists; highly recommended.

Team Sports (indoor or outdoor)

Good for voice: Fitness, stress management, teamwork.

Cautions and comments: Limit shouting, yelling, cheering, coaching. You're a vocal athlete, too, and you have to be true to that discipline as well as your sport. Limit alcohol and talking over noise at postgame parties.

Yoga

Good for voice: Fully expansive breathing, mindfulness and subtle-body awareness, relaxation, posture and balance, flexibility, unity of body-mind-breath.

Cautions and comments: As in any fitness activity, learn to manage your breath without closing the throat. If you commonly exhale with a sudden explosion, inhale less air and soften the entire practice.

Deliberately constricted, audible *Ujjayi* breathing can be stressful to the voice if the constriction is placed low in the throat. If you practice this technique, protect your voice by focusing the turbulence and heat of Ujjayi closer to the soft palate. When in doubt, keep your breathing silent to protect vocal folds from air turbulence, dryness, and fatigue.

The Headstand, Shoulderstand, Plough, Fish, and similar poses that emphasize the neck should be avoided after any kind of vocal surgery. Wait at least a month or until your doctor says it is safe to return to them.

See References for my article on yoga and voice, including more comments on breath adjustments.

The five S's of sports training are: stamina, speed, strength, skill, and spirit; but the greatest of these is spirit.

—Ken Doherty

Chapter 9 Summary

- Physical fitness and exercise support your vocal health, with a few adjustments.

- Emphasize activities that build cardiovascular fitness and flexibility, and that enhance your awareness of posture and energy flow.

- If you lift weights or do other strength-building activities, be very careful to keep your throat, neck, and breathing relaxed.

- Limit yelling and cheering that may strain your voice.

- Stay hydrated.

- Think of voice use as a kind of internal athletics.

10

Warming Up the Voice

Students often ask for "warm-up tips" or what I would call a "recipe" for warming up. Nobody ever asks what a warm-up is supposed to achieve.
—Alexander Massey

Warming up the voice is not the same as practicing. Warming up for any physical or mental activity is a process of physiological and mental preparation. Warm-up exercises get you ready to practice.

Because the vocal mechanism is so deeply internal and the rest of your process requires a special kind of self-awareness, the first step of any warm-up must be to turn your attention inward. Shift the mind from external distractions to self-curiosity: for example, "How am I doing today?"

Your mood and general physical state are important to notice for several reasons. If you'll be doing a longer practice session, knowing whether you feel superenergetic or definitely tired or blue may influence how long you spend and what goals you set for the rest of your vocal session. Pushing to get those high notes even if your body just isn't up to it today—or working to exhaustion because you feel super-great or superupset—will get in the way of steady progress. You can't avoid those temptations until you know where they live.

Most important, though, is the inescapable fact that your body sensations and emotions are tied together, and both are wired into your voice. Allowing mood or pain signals into your consciousness is the only way to be sure you're feeling your body fully—and that's the most important thing for vocal safety.

A warm-up should aim to heighten the singer's awareness of what the different muscle groups are doing and how they are interacting in the act of making vocal sounds . . . unless we can do this, we have little chance of doing [other warm-ups] well. Does everything feel alert but easy, and does the mind feel calm and aware, rather than "revved up," narrowly focused on sound, one muscle group, or something extraneous? . . . We must answer with intuition, with whole self and "felt sense." "Thinking" too hard narrows our awareness and takes it away from whole-self/body-consciousness.

—Alexander Massey

After this mental check-in, the next step is to wake up the body. If your life is generally sedentary, start your voice session with a few minutes of light aerobics, yoga, tai chi, or simple range-of-motion exercises like head-neck circles, shoulder circles, torso twists and hip circles. On the other hand, if you're generally on the go, slow yoga postures and breathing exercises might be a better contrast and more helpful for balancing your attention.

Fitzmaurice Voicework, my current foundation, is a dynamic yet relaxing process that prepares the body for sound using specialized body and breath exercises that simultaneously build energy, awareness, relaxation, and freedom. See the website list in the "References and Suggested Reading" chapter at the end of this book for more information.

Developing the Vibration

From here, a typical vocal warm-up would use easy humming, tongue trills, or lip trills (sometimes called lip bubbles—what brass players do, or kids mimicking engine noises). Keep your sounds medium quiet at first, even a little breathy. Catherine Fitzmaurice calls this "fluffy sound," emphasizing a generous, but not forced, use of air. Keep your body moving as you loosen up the voice; stretch your face and tongue, energize the mouth, and yawn.

If you have learned how to enhance the resonance or "placement" of vibrations in your face, begin to bring those tones into your voice too, while keeping your throat easy and comfortable. Sometimes a light *zzzzz* is fun, or a modified hum on *nnn* or *ng*. Use whatever sound gives you the most buzzy vibration feelings in your mouth and face without having to push or force at all.

Another very comfortable warm-up is to use a drinking straw as you would a kazoo: pucker around the straw as if it's an extension of your lips on an exaggerated vowel *ooo*. Vocalize on that long *ooo* vowel in your middle and upper ranges, staying relaxed in your throat and sending the sound through the straw.

This can look or feel a little goofy, but it's actually a very healthy exercise that helps the vocal folds move freely, and it feels round and warm inside the throat. For more instruction, look at Ingo Titze's

YouTube videos on vocalizing with a straw.

According to voice scientists, the healthiest production feels easy, comfortable, and effortless in the throat and resonant or vibrant in the face. So for vocal health and safety, those are the feelings to aim for in your warm-up.

If you're in doubt about how much to do on a given day (Are you getting sick? Extra tired? Just imagining problems?), try singing or talking in a high and soft register. This is physiologically the hardest thing for you to do with your voice, so it tests your outer limits. For more detail, look online for the "swelling tests," as developed by Dr. Robert Bastian, Marina Gilman, and others.

Five to ten minutes of preparing your mind, body, and breath, plus five minutes of easy, resonant vocalizing can be an adequate vocal warm-up, if performed regularly. From there, you're ready to practice deeper aspects of technique, develop new material, or

Online Forum Question from a Rock Singer

Rock singer: The doctor says I have swollen, irregular vocal cords, and that's why I sound raspy when I talk. But if I scream or sing really loud for an hour or so, I sound fine! When we have a road gig, I just go outside in the parking lot after soundcheck and yell until my voice clears up. What's wrong with that?

My answer: Vigorous vocalizing with the aggressive technique you describe can make the soft outer layers of your vocal cords temporarily swell up. Extra fluid and blood are drawn in because your cords are getting bruised. That swelling might temporarily fill in or smooth over the chronic irregularities at the vocal edges that make you sound raspy. Afterward, your vocal folds might seem to meet more easily with a clearer sound.

But your instrument will not be happy inside. Your pitch range will be even more limited. You won't be able to make soft sounds, and you'll face the public. If you're about to go onstage, just add a quick review of your opening or any important names to pronounce.

Once you're familiar with good technique, a healthy, well-balanced voice should be available without a lot of effort. So if you find that you need a long warm-up to get your voice where you want it, something may be wrong.

be very hoarse by the end of the show. The next day, you will sound worse rather than better. If the doctor looked at your cords again, they'd be red and even more irregular at the edges. You've gotten through one gig while risking permanent damage.

Whipping a horse may make him run fast, but not forever. This approach is not recommended if you want a long career.

Cooling Down

Athletic training often includes a cooldown period that is the inverse or "bookend" of warming up. This practice allows the body to return to a resting level with minimum strain and allows your metabolism to begin "taking out the trash" left over from vigorous muscular effort.

Although cooling down vocally gets discussed from time to time within the training and rehabilitation communities, there isn't any re-search yet on what, if any, activities do the best job. The recipe that follows is my own speculation, a set of practices that are known to be safe, generally supportive to vocal health, and that therefore make sense in a cooldown process. Try them and see how they work for you.

Vocally, use the light exercises that began your warm-up: lip buzz-es, tongue trills, humming, zzzzz, or the straw kazoo. Any whole-body stretching that you used as a warm-up can be repeated at a gentle pace to cool down your whole system. Massage the throat (on and around the voice box), neck, and jaw-muscle areas, and add yawns and tongue stretches to ease the throat muscles.

A hot shower or other steam treatment when you get home helps relieve the immediate surface wear and tear on the edges of the vocal cords. Slowing the breath and bringing your mental focus to present time (you're not onstage any more) will help prepare your body for restorative sleep.

> Whatever is flexible and flowing will tend to grow;
> whatever is rigid and blocked will wither and die.
> **—Tao Te Ching**

Chapter 10 Summary

- When it's time to warm up your voice, stop other activities and make a conscious choice to clear your mind of past or future tasks. Turn your attention to the present.

- Have some water or tea nearby and sip throughout the warm-up.

- Do a few minutes of body movement, be it vigorous, slow and relaxing, or a combination of both. Focus on the sensations of your body and breath, and allow your emotional mood to be in your awareness but not overwhelming.

- Begin to make easy sounds with light trills of your lips, tongue, *zzzz* buzz, humming, or using a straw. Slide comfortably through your pitch range, staying soft or medium soft. Gradually make the sounds louder and use a wider pitch range.

- If your voice feels tired or effortful, alternate silent body or breath exercises with vocal ones. Stay attentive to process and sensation, not result.

- After 5 to 10 minutes, you are warmed up and ready to practice specific techniques or material, or to perform or present what you have rehearsed in prior sessions.

- If these guidelines seem too vague or mysterious to you, look for a voice class at a college drama or theater department, professional theater company, or acting studio; I consider these the best sources of basic warm-ups for all kinds of voice use. For further information, see chapter 23, "Training."

- Use similar activities and self-massage or steam as a cooldown process after your performance, presentation, or practice session.

Intervention: Vocal Health Care

Health is a dynamic and harmonious equilibrium
of all the elements and forces making up
and surrounding a human being.
—Andrew Weil, MD

To keep the body in good health is a duty . . . otherwise
we shall not be able to keep our mind strong and clear.
—Buddha

Be careful about reading health books.
You may die of a misprint.
—Mark Twain

11

First Aid for Hoarseness

Did you spend the weekend partying over noise? Did you shout to someone for help and feel vocally rough afterward? If this happens regularly, there's a bigger problem, but if your voice is generally healthy and flexible, here's a recovery recipe. Consider it a single-use package.

1. Rest the voice as much as possible for 48 to 72 hours. *Seriously*—no singing or talking, except for the exercises in item 4, below.

2. Drink 2 quarts or liters of water or tea per day, or 3 quarts or liters if you're a large person. Ingest absolutely no alcohol or coffee or anything you are even mildly allergic to.

3. Breathe (plain) steam for 5 to 10 minutes, 1 to 2 times each day, as described in chapter 5, "Air."

4. For 1 to 2 minutes every hour or two throughout the day, use one of the following exercises. Choose one or the other or alternate. These are physiologically the safest types of vocalizing and may help cellular healing, similar to the warm-ups mentioned in chapter 10, but they are done for a shorter time. Permitted exercises are the following:

   a. Light, easy humming on a medium tone or on pitch glides up and down, with a very nasal or buzzy feeling in the front of the face.

   b. Light, easy-quality *oooh* through a straw in medium- to high-pitch range.

Do not force the voice. If it's hard to make sound, stay quiet. Skip this vocal step entirely if you lost your voice very suddenly, or if your doctor has diagnosed a vocal-cord hemorrhage or high risk for one. Such conditions need complete vocal rest, and a diagnostic throat exam if you haven't had one yet.

5. No weight lifting or heavy labor that involves holding your breath *at all*. Go easy on abdominal workouts, too, unless you're really good at not holding your breath when you crunch.

6. Maximum self-care in general: light healthy meals, moderate exercise, prayer or meditation, massage or bodywork, and good sleep.

7. See the best laryngologist you can afford if you experience any of the following:

   a. Your voice disappears in an instant, or

   b. You feel pain in your voice or throat, or

c. There is no improvement in 2 to 3 days, or

d. Your voice doesn't return to normal in 10 to 14 days, or

e. You can force your voice to sound normal again, but you
   secretly know it isn't!

Everyone wants a magic pill to make hoarseness disappear. All you can do is make problems disappear from your future life—by preventing them before they start. So use the vocal time-out to reread this book and its resources. Meditate on your ability to take better care of yourself, set limits on vocal demands, and protect your fabulous—but not infinite—voice from now on. It's also a good time to use my *Visualizations for Singers* CD (see my website, The Voice of Your Life, at www.voiceofyourlife.com).

Don't speak unless you can improve on the silence.
—Spanish proverb

Chapter 11 Summary

- After extreme voice use, give your throat a few days
  of special care.

- Emphasize silence, moisture, and brief, gentle warm-up
  exercises.

- If you stay hoarse, don't wait more than two weeks
  before seeing an ear-nose-throat doctor.

- Learn from the experience in order to prevent problems
  in the future.

12

Seeing a Doctor

*The office of medicine is but to tune this curious harp
of man's body and to reduce it to harmony.*
—Sir Francis Bacon

Why a Throat Exam Is Important

There are now many websites with extensive information on medical voice care. These sites are great for educating yourself about the vocal instrument. But voice problems cannot be diagnosed or judged accurately by sound or by how your throat feels to you.

Remember that when the voice works well, you don't feel anything at all. Changes in the sound or comfort of your voice—hoarseness, pain, or fatigue—are important to notice as signs that something might be wrong. However, these altered sounds or sensations are vague indicators; the same huskiness could be simple overuse, a cold, or cancer.

Hoarseness is usually not cancer—I'm not trying to scare you here. My point is that a specific voice diagnosis and the best treatment plan for the diagnosis are impossible to know without having a doctor's exam that includes looking (indirectly) at your vocal cords.

> If you trust Google more than your doctor,
> then maybe it's time to switch doctors.
> **—Jadelr and Cristina Cordova**

When to See a Doctor

Hans von Leden, MD, one of the fathers of vocal-arts medicine, explains in his many lectures that there are four main reasons to go to a doctor for a throat exam:

1. Hoarseness or other change in the sound or ease of the voice that lasts more than two weeks

2. Pain associated with using the voice

3. Sudden loss of voice or other sudden change, especially during a performance

4. Lack of normal progress in voice training, as judged by the teacher in comparison to other similar students

Even if nothing is wrong, in the best of all possible worlds, every serious vocal artist would get a laryngeal checkup every year.

Which Doctor to Choose

Your quest for medical voice care may begin with a visit to your primary or general-practice doctor. This visit is required by some insurance plans, but it may not be necessary once you have a relationship with a voice specialist. You might instead start with an ear-nose-throat physician (ENT, or *otolaryngologist*), someone with more expertise in this whole area of the body than a general practitioner.

Within the ENT field, however, voice medicine (*laryngology*) has now developed as a small, more detailed subspecialty. If you use your voice heavily or professionally, this is the type of specialist you should seek out.

Laryngologists who are especially interested in voice are often singers themselves, or are otherwise involved with music. They have probably sought advanced training at a major research center, they are most likely to have invested in good diagnostic equipment, and they stay up to date by attending the professional conferences at which the special problems of singers, lecturers, and other voice performers are investigated and discussed.

But note that the doctor whom "all the singers go to" may not always be the most knowledgeable. You want to see the doctor that the *healthiest* singers go to! The best voice clinics also offer a team approach to care, where patients are seen by an MD, speech pathologist, and perhaps other practitioners such as a psychologist, singing specialist, or physical therapist when appropriate.

A national online directory of well-respected clinics for vocal artists is included in the "References and Suggested Reading" section at the end of this book. Specialty voice clinics like this are not yet established widely enough to serve all of the vocalists who need care. Start where you can, and contact one of the major centers in your region to ask about individual specialists who may be more accessible to you.

What to Expect When You Go

Currently, the most advanced type of voice exam is called *video-stroboscopy*. An endoscope is inserted through the nose (known as a "flexible scope") or placed into the mouth (a "rigid" or "fixed scope"). These small tubes have either a fiber-optic lens and light attached to a small camera or a digital-camera chip built in. A strobe light attached to these instruments provides a slow-motion view of the vocal folds in motion.

Not all laryngologists or other ENT doctors have invested in this equipment, especially in rural areas or at facilities that are not part of a university or research center. Doctors without videostrobe equipment may be wise and well meaning, but they will have a harder time making a correct diagnosis.

A 2001 review by Leonard and Kendall of voice patients examined with and without videostroboscopy showed that the nonstrobe diagnoses were correct only about a third of the time. A third of the cases reviewed with stroboscopy showed the original diagnosis plus an additional problem, and a third had completely different findings.

If you are serious about voice use but you live in a more remote location, try to save up for travel to a specialty clinic. Diagnosis and treatment by a less-experienced doctor or without videostrobe equipment may be incomplete and can cost you more in the long run in extended work problems or personal frustration.

There are no good substitutes for a visual exam with videostroboscopy and a laryngologist who is familiar with the needs of vocalists and who stays up-to-date at conferences on voice medicine.

If health insurance is a problem, try to save money when you are healthy so you can get voice care when you need it. Talk frankly to the doctors whom you consult; some will adjust their rates for vocal artists in need.

What Happens After the Exam

Treatment by a laryngologist typically involves some combination of medication, referral to speech therapy, and in some cases, surgery. If there is any question about treatment, or if vocal surgery is discussed, consider getting a second opinion with the best-credentialed specialist you can find.

Understanding Your Reluctance

There is some interesting new research about singers who avoid seeking medical help. For classical singers, the main obstacles appear to be medical costs and difficulty taking time off. Pop, musical theater, and other performers share these problems. But one study showed that they are less likely to seek help for voice problems than for other health concerns!

Why would a serious voice user spend time and money on other health issues and still neglect the voice? Is there a lack of trust in medical care? Hopefully this book, and other education, will show that good clinics exist, staffed by physicians and allied professionals who genuinely know and care about vocal health. Voice medicine is a young field, but it's maturing fast.

What about desire to deny there's a problem? Fear of being thought a "diva" for not just muscling through? If talent is supposed to overcome trouble, do signs of trouble mean one has insufficient talent? Perhaps it's better not to find out.

Maybe treating the "magical" voice as a normal organ that deserves regular checkups and care just ruins the mystique. Or is there something even deeper at work? The public image of the artist, of course, is of someone tortured as well as glamorous, self-destructive as well as self-promoting. Might as well neglect your throats (or smoke and drink too much). The artist's life is hard enough that one is expected to run hard and fail young.

This attitude reveals the opposite of the glamorous view—a notion that artists are worth very little, that they are disposable. The term *talent*, after all, is used by casting directors to refer to performers in general, especially to the throngs of "wannabes" ready to replace anyone who fails. Do vocalists internalize this disrespect and stay away from the doctor because they don't believe they deserve care?

I've glimpsed many of these attitudes in my clients, and I know that my research-minded colleagues are working to understand them better. A decision to seek health care (or not) is very private, and not always conscious—kind of like the larynx itself.

Let me just reinforce the perspective of my opening chapters. The power of the voice may always be somewhat mysterious, but its mechanics are less and less so. We're not in the dark ages anymore.

Preventative care will go a long way. It is best matched by an ongoing relationship with a good laryngologist who can reassure you about minor problems and actively help with more serious ones. Every human being with a voice deserves this care.

> I am not afraid of storms for I am
> learning how to sail my ship.
> **—Louisa May Alcott**

Chapter 12 Summary

- When you are healthy, locate the best cross-disciplinary voice clinic(s) in your region and save up some money in advance so that you can get a good exam when you need one.

- See a medical voice specialist (laryngologist) if you experience throat pain, sudden changes in your voice, lingering hoarseness or cough without other symptoms, or if your voice teacher suggests it.

- Don't spend too much time trying to figure out what's wrong by focusing tightly on how you sound or how your throat feels. General self-education is great, but when things go wrong, the changes you feel or hear are not specific enough for a diagnosis.

- Don't try to diagnose yourself online. No blogger has the exact same anatomy, health history, or combination of risks as you.

- Voice problems are not usually serious, but they can be complex and subtle.

- A visual examination with videostroboscopy, combined with a thorough clinical interview, is the best current diagnostic approach.

- Your best medical treatment depends on the diagnosis and on your individual situation.

- If you love your voice, give it the best care you can.

13

Complementary and Alternative Medicine

A Short History of Medicine
2000 BC—"Here, eat this root."
1000 BC—"That root is heathen. Say this prayer."
AD 1850—"That prayer is superstition. Drink this potion."
AD 1940—"That potion is snake oil. Swallow this pill."
AD 1985—"That pill is ineffective. Take this antibiotic."
AD 2000—"That antibiotic is artificial. Here, eat this root."
—**Author unknown**

News reports show that in the United States, people now use "alternative" remedies and procedures as often—or even more often—than mainstream medicine. A philosophical preference for "natural" versus "synthetic" ingredients, distrust of institutional- and pharmaceutical-based care, frustration over costs and insurance coverage, and interest in mind-body interactions all increase the appeal of accessible systems linked to traditional cultures and of do-it-yourself remedies.

Similar studies also indicate that the people who use alternative remedies rarely discuss them with their mainstream physician. Fortunately, a slowly growing number of health-care providers, specialists, and researchers use both mainstream and alternative techniques, an approach called "integrative" or "complementary-alternative medicine" (CAM). Recent changes in the funding of health-care research and the open-mindedness of younger medical researchers are improving our knowledge about how well alternative-health practices actually work and for what conditions.

Some laryngologists include CAM in their recommendations, and in time there will surely be more crossover knowledge to help voice users of all cultural backgrounds and lifestyle preferences.

Everything on the earth has a purpose, every disease an herb to cure it, and every person a mission.
—Mourning Dove, Salish People

Balancing the Benefits

As a broad generalization, mainstream medicine may be best at diagnosis: determining and naming what is wrong. Laryngeal technologies—fiber-optic scopes and the like—have identified and differentiated voice problems that most other healing systems approach as generic "hoarseness" or "sore throat." For instance, only a high-tech voice exam can distinguish between throat tension as a primary problem and excess tension by which someone compensates for an underlying vocal weakness. Mainstream treatments are similarly diagnosis-specific and symptom-related.

Alternative approaches, often termed *whole-person* or *holistic*, are more likely to examine or treat many aspects of the person and lifestyle, and their benefits may be slower or more subtle. This is appropriate for some kinds of voice complaints, but it can also be frustratingly nonspecific. Once again, the field of voice seems to be unique, in that good treatment can demand a combination of methods—neither the close-up, cellular-level view nor the big-picture, mind-body view seem fully adequate.

So one complementary or integrative approach to vocal health care would be to see an experienced laryngologist to diagnose your voice problems and follow the doctor's recommendations to recover from the immediate problem. In addition, explore more holistic, non-mainstream methods to support or deepen your healing process and prevent future lapses.

In this small health guide, it is impossible to review all the possible benefits and risks of the many alternative or non-Western health-care practices and practitioners. I personally use some herbal remedies and receive occasional chiropractic and acupuncture treatments along with prescription medicines and appropriate medical checkups. But I am wary about recommending the same to patients, except in general terms, because I'm licensed to provide only speech therapy.

Sound Mind, Sound Body

The stories of mind-body medicine . . . knit together domains of experience that we struggle otherwise to relate: the medical and the moral, the biological and the biographical, the natural and the cultural.

—Anne Harrington

When we are highly stressed, depressed, anxious, or pessimistic and convinced of our powerlessness, our bodies are less resistant to illness and less able to repair the normal wear and tear of daily life. The voice bears the same health risks as other cells and organs. If we are under chronic stress, not sleeping well, coping with changing relationships, or afraid of losing a job, the body's mechanisms for routine repair, cellular maintenance, and immune responses to infection may be compromised.

Optimism, a reliable family or social network, and some type of private contemplation, have all been proven to benefit the body in measurable ways. There is even research evidence that people recover from colds more quickly if they feel compassion and personal caring from their doctor!

Nevertheless, the narrow, cell-and-molecule emphasis of mainstream medicine leads to criticism that physicians may not routinely address the connections between vocal function and other aspects of the body, mind, and emotions. In fact, the best laryngologists I know do acknowledge that stress and other psychological factors are often wrapped into voice problems.

When their own time with patients is constrained, these doctors appreciate speech therapists and healthy-voice trainers and teachers who incorporate thoughtful and relevant counseling techniques. These practices may help voice users by reducing anxiety, reducing the internal distress when vocal difficulties arise, and helping people to stay hopeful during the course of medical treatment.

A few years ago, I chatted with a young ENT at a medical voice conference. He said to me, "People come to my office, and I look at them and examine their throats. Sometimes I think, 'This person needs an antibiotic.' But I'm also thinking that he or she needs [to do] pranayama [yoga breathing exercises] to help relax and manage stress. I can't just tell them that but then send them away with their prescription for an antibiotic. I want to offer what I know will really make them better in the long run. So now that I've finished my clinical fellowship, I'm studying to be a yoga teacher."

Integrative Medicine

Drugs are not always necessary.
Belief in recovery always is.
—Norman Cousins

If you use alternative therapies, especially herbal remedies, tell your physician about them to avoid negative or unexpected interactions between the two medical systems. These concerns can be real chemistry, not just prejudice.

Similarly, if you choose some mainstream care, avoid alternative practitioners who fear or aggressively criticize what you're doing. Open-mindedness is an important ingredient on all sides of the healing arts.

Subconscious beliefs about healing systems—and about yourself—have been shown to have a strong influence on whether any treatment is effective. Whether you choose mainstream care, alternative care, or a combination of both, you are most likely to receive lasting benefit from a health-care approach that you believe in and that is offered by a doctor or healer with whom you feel comfortable.

Chapter 13 Summary

- Many alternative and mind-body health practices may be useful for general wellness, stress relief, healthy digestion, and so on, and thus contribute to preventative voice care.

- Few nonmainstream health systems demonstrate a thorough understanding of vocal function, nor do they offer the diagnostic precision of modern laryngology for acute conditions.

- An integrative, combined approach may best serve your vocal health.

- Both laryngologists and alternative practitioners may be uncomfortable with a combination of modalities, so be aware of prejudices on all sides.

- Intuitively trusting your body about your overall health is often helpful. But as repeated throughout this book, in relation to something specific in your throat, inner senses may not be quite as reliable as you'd like.

- Nevertheless, all kinds of treatments tend to work better when people believe in them.

- Stay tuned as the fields of both laryngology and integrative medicine continue to evolve.

14

Speech Therapy for Voice Problems

She sells seashells by the seashore. The rest of the year, she's a speech pathologist.
—Author unknown

If you have a voice problem related to how, or how much, you use your voice, or if other medical conditions have caused changes in your voice that muscle retraining can help resolve, your laryngologist may refer you to a speech pathologist (less formally called a speech therapist). Think of this as physical therapy for your throat.

Just as not all ENTs are true laryngologists, not all speech pathologists have a thorough, up-to-date understanding of the voice and voice therapy. It is a small subspecialty within the profession. As with your efforts to find a voice-knowledgeable doctor, finding a voice-rehabilitation specialist may mean traveling farther or going "out of network." If your voice is a primary tool of your trade, or otherwise central to your personal identity, these efforts may spare you time, work, and frustration in the long run.

In true voice clinics staffed by a multidisciplinary team, the speech pathologist may perform an initial videostroboscopic exam (described in chapter 12, "Seeing a Doctor") and review the results with the laryngologist. Or they may both be present from the outset.

Whereas a doctor examines your vocal cords to look for specific cell changes (*lesions*) such as nodules, swelling, or inflammation, the speech pathologist focuses on how the cords are working: how they move in and out of vibratory position; whether the vibration is complete and fluid or is irregular, interrupted in some small area; and how the surrounding muscles behave.

The speech pathologist will also talk with you about the demands on your voice, your general health, and your vocal habits, and will record and analyze your vocal sound. Some speech pathologists also measure airflow using a special mask while you sing or talk. The review of your personal and medical history may uncover contributing factors that you thought were unrelated to the throat.

Simple Goals

Once there is a clear picture of the factors that have contributed to the problem—and often there are several—you'll discuss treatment. The goals of speech therapy are to help resolve the current problem and to protect you from future trouble using behavioral, educational, and counseling approaches alongside the doctor's tools of medication and so on.

The speech pathologist may suggest lifestyle adjustments, including many issues addressed in this book, and will develop an individualized plan of exercises to retrain your voice. He or she will work with you to rehabilitate weaknesses; train efficient, effective voice technique for your needs; troubleshoot specific voice situations; and establish healthy vocal habits for the long term.

Voice-rehabilitation services are typically offered in a 4- to 12-week timeframe. They may be covered by medical insurance, depending on your individual plan and situation. When the therapy program is complete, you may "graduate" from care and be referred back to your singing teachers, to another voice specialist, or to a class or community group.

What a License Means

Some aspects of speech therapy can be similar to working with a singing or speech coach. However, there are important differences.

A speech pathologist is formally licensed, meeting certain standards of medical and scientific knowledge. Speech pathologists are required to stay up to date through continuing education at conferences and seminars, and we are held accountable for the quality of care we provide with multiple levels of review.

Artistic voice teachers are often very skilled and insightful, but at present they are not legally qualified to work with damaged voices, except in collaboration with a medical team. Some vocal-arts teachers protest this delineation and advertise rehabilitation services. As someone working under a regulated license and answerable to a code of medical ethics and other layers of supervision, I can't fully support those who disrespect such safeguards.

Some turf disagreements are unavoidable, as between other close-ly related professions. Our different voice professions continue to evolve, interact, cross-train, and gradually understand each other's perspectives. Our networks are young, as is the entire voice field, but they are developing internationally.

In the best situation, you are seen by a speech pathologist who has training in the vocal arts or works closely with an artistic voice coach as well as with the laryngologist. An official statement on such collaboration follows.

The Role of the Speech-Language Pathologist, the Teacher of Singing, and the Speaking Voice Trainer in Voice Rehabilitation

Since the founding of the American Speech-Language-Hearing Association (ASHA) in 1925, the founding of the National Association of Teachers of Singing (NATS) in 1944, and the founding of the Voice and Speech Trainers Association (VASTA) in 1986, there has been increasing awareness of (a) the importance of having healthy laryngeal function in all styles of speech and singing and (b) the existence of a connection between optimal vocal usage in speech and optimal vocal usage in singing.

All three organizations acknowledge that the most effective path to vocal recovery often will include an integrated approach to optimal voice care and production that addresses both speech and singing tasks. ASHA, NATS, and VASTA therefore collectively affirm the importance of interdisciplinary management of speakers and singers with voice problems and disorders, with the management team ideally consisting of some or all of the following individuals: an otolaryngologist, a speech-language pathologist, and a singing teacher and/or speaking voice and speech trainer...

ASHA, NATS, and VASTA encourage their members to cooperate in the development and delivery of interdisciplinary programs and services for singers and other professional voice users with voice disorders.

—*Excerpted from* American Speech-Language-Hearing Association Technical Report *(see www.asha.org/docs/html/ TR2005-00147.html)*

Chapter 14 Summary

- The terms *speech therapist, speech pathologist,* and *speech-language pathologist* all refer to the same profession.

- Speech pathologists without specialty training can treat simple voice problems; vocal artists and professional speakers are best served at clinics known for voice expertise.

- Therapy for vocal injuries typically involves both technical exercises and lifestyle counseling.

- Singing teachers who offer to rehabilitate vocal injuries are not licensed to do so and are not supervised or legally accountable for their services.

15

Coping with Colds

Not everything is based on Karma. Whether you lead a good life or a bad one, exposure to pathogenic microbes can still make you sick.
—Vianna Stibal

Cold symptoms do not result from the destructive effects of viruses but from the body's response to these intruders.
—Jennifer Ackerman

In medical jargon, the common cold is called an *upper respiratory infection*, or URI. Serious voice users have the same risk as anyone else for picking up these annoying bugs. But for us, the consequences are more severe, especially if the infection gets into the throat.

How exactly does a cold hurt your voice? Actually, it's the body's reaction to the cold virus that causes problems. When the virus invades the lining of your nose, mouth, and throat, your body sends extra fluid, blood, and immune-system cells to the area. That's why these areas get swollen.

Swollen vocal folds vibrate more slowly, which makes vocal pitch shift lower. The folds may also vibrate unevenly, or "leak air" between slightly irregular edges, leading you to sound hoarse, rough, or raspy. Other vocal symptoms of a URI can include a smaller pitch range, especially the loss of high notes (bulkier cords don't stretch as far) and less control over loudness (that all-or-nothing honk).

Extra congestion in the nose or sinuses can block resonance, making your voice sound dull. Chest congestion or overall fatigue can hurt your breath support. Repeated coughing can irritate otherwise healthy vocal fords.

Under any of these conditions, pushing or tensing to try to sound "normal" will give you more trouble in the long run. Instead, as discussed in chapter 11, "First Aid for Hoarseness," a few days of relative silence—plus sleep, fluids, and steam—will help your voice to recover quickly and help you to avoid compromising your vocal technique.

Dr. Neil Schachter's book, *The Good Doctor's Guide to Colds and Flu*, is full of great information and advice (see the chapter at the end of this book called "References and Suggested Reading"). He recommends the following:

- To keep from getting colds, wash your hands often, and use antimicrobial cleaning sprays on common surfaces and objects.

- At the first sign of a cold, take 500 mg of vitamin C daily; also helpful are zinc nasal spray or swabs, and (yes) chicken soup. As symptoms develop or linger, continue the above, plus a glass of orange juice every day, hot tea, and plenty of other fluids. Take a hot shower every

morning to loosen phlegm. Twice per day, use warm
water and a bit of salt to gargle (for sore throat)
or rinse your nasal passages.

- Use a vaporizer or humidifier during the night. Eat light
meals for the first few days you are ill. Use over-the-counter remedies for symptomatic relief. Resume a normal diet
after a few days.

- If all symptoms are above the neck, it is safe to continue
your regular fitness routines. If symptoms involve your
chest, take a few days off from vigorous exercise.

- Call your regular doctor if you have trouble breathing,
chest pain, or a fever of 102 degrees (F) or higher.

Jennifer Ackerman's book, *Ah-Choo: The Uncommon Life of Your Common Cold*, reinforces Schachter's emphasis on prevention, but casts more doubt on cold remedies in general. Zinc and vitamin C, she contends, are useful only for those in extreme circumstances, such as prisoners of war or soldiers in the Arctic.

Ackerman agrees that there is no better prevention than washing your hands frequently, especially when traveling or meeting lots of people. During cold season or when others are ill, frequently clean things that everyone touches, such as doorknobs and faucets, micro-wave-oven controls, and telephones of all kinds.

For symptom relief, Ackerman smartly recommends over-the-counter cold remedies with single ingredients, rather than cover-the-bases formulas with multiple ingredients. For example, if you're congested, use decongestants and antihistamines; if achy, an anti-inflammatory; if coughing, an expectorant. This approach minimizes unwanted side effects and helps you think strategically about your body and its messages.

Ackerman is especially critical of the use of so-called immune boosters like echinacea. If most of a cold's misery comes from the body's immune response, she suggests that after the cold starts, increasing the cellular drama waged by your immune system might just make you more miserable! Treated or untreated, the typical cold lasts about a week.

Paying attention to your health when you're feeling well—with good habits of nutrition, exercise, rest, and social support—is the deeper process recommended throughout this book, and it will pay off in fewer, lighter colds and flu.

What Do I Put in My Tea?

Tea has earned a reputation as something to drink when you have a cold. Green tea has gotten a lot of praise recently for antioxidant properties. Regular (black) tea turns out to have just as many helpful ingredients, and it is somewhat better at relieving chest congestion.

Any hot beverage, including plain hot water, can help keep you hydrated, thin out secretions (phlegm), increase circulation in the throat, and send steamy vapors into the airway.

Neither lemon nor honey has been proven to have any particular benefits for the common cold, but they are not harmful either. Use them to taste.

A formula of slippery elm tea was formally studied in people with colds and sore throat. It relieved more discomfort than the "placebo" tea in the comparison, but only for about 30 minutes. Many singers favor ginger tea, which warms the throat and eases digestion.

The only way to treat the common cold is with contempt.
—Sir William Osler

If the Show Must Go On

If you simultaneously have a cold and a commitment to sing or speak in public, the dilemma can be more difficult than your fogged-in brain wants to deal with. Canceling or postponing your audition, show, or presentation may seem to put at risk your career, school grade, management, friendships, or loyalty to a director. Trying to sound your best with inflamed or painful vocal cords may risk doing further damage to them.

Common lore advises that established stars and beginners have the most freedom to cancel an appearance without serous consequences. Those at the middle stages of a career or training program are under the most scrutiny and most at risk for being judged unreliable, unavailable, or inadequate.

For all voice users, these dilemmas spotlight the importance of a relationship with a doctor and therapy or training team whom you know and trust, a relationship established before the crisis hits. Talk with these folks honestly about whether you are risking further vocal damage if you push yourself to perform and about balancing the health and professional risks.

There are prescription medications that some physicians offer that can knock back the effects of an acute laryngeal inflammation in time for an important performance. But don't push your luck by constantly talking, singing, preaching, or shouting when ill.

If you decide to go on, rehearse in shorter sessions, and be extra attentive to your vocal technique. Respect any temporary limits on your pitch range, tone quality, or breathing. Maintain the emotional connection to your material, and communicate that meaning even if your sound is less than you hope for.

Drink plenty of fluids and be especially cautious about exposure to smoke, hairspray, or other irritants. Minimize nonessential talking (such as backstage chatter or extended verbal agonizing about how to handle your illness).

If you need to meet and greet guests before or after the show, stay at the edge of the crowd (less background noise), smile more than you speak, and keep water or tea with you. Shower or steam after the show, before you go to sleep.

The Temptations

I have worked with high-level performing artists who admit that when illness strikes, they tend to repeatedly "test" their voice on the hardest bits of material. This stresses the voice, reinforces habits of tension and anxiety, and disrupts their familiar preparation routine.

It is far better to rest as much as you can, then do a normal but extramindful preparation process in warm-up and rehearsal, even if the result is not perfect. Pushing yourself to sound normal before you are completely healthy increases the risk of doing permanent vocal damage. More commonly, there is a risk of falling into bad habits of tension and other compensations that will be hard to unlearn.

Many voice patients whom I see in the spring or summer trace their problems back to the winter holiday season, when they got a bad cold, became exhausted, but sang or talked a lot anyway. Vocalizing with swollen cords and reduced breath support required extra effort and tension, which then became ingrained bad habits.

Six or eight months down the road, these patients found they had deeper voice problems, more anxiety, and larger medical bills that could have been avoided. So even during periods of heavy vocal demand, do your best to pay attention to early warning signs and plan ahead accordingly.

Personal Note: Colds

As a child, I got frequent colds and suffered strep throat once or twice every year. I spent one winter of college with endless bronchitis, singing in the choir as if padded by phlegm everywhere. I was tested for allergies, but avoiding the reported allergens didn't make much difference, nor did a tonsillectomy in my senior year.

I continued to struggle with recurrent colds and congestion through decades as a yoga-intense vegetarian, advanced theater student, political activist, and aspiring musician. I had to cancel one major concert associated with a CD launch due to illness—but the alternative would have been to sound really bad! I was barely comforted when a bad storm hit that night, keeping most of the audience home anyway.

Over many years, I have come to understand my best individual nutritional plan, and I've found my way through many levels of emotional and spiritual healing. Colds and related infections have gradually become less frequent and less severe. Recently, even when bad flu and cold bugs hit many of my clients, I've noticed that I stay immune.

It's been a very long process, and there are still viruses out there that will get to me. I'm definitely fortunate to have access to good food, a generally secure life, and good medical care of both mainstream and natural kinds. I don't take these circumstances for granted.

My main point is that self-care is a process, and it is very individual, not a same-for-everyone prescription. Do your best, find your way, and keep learning what works for you.

Chapter 15 Summary

- Prevention remains your best defense against colds; be diligent.

- The components of general wellness—the by-now-boring basics of nutrition, sleep, exercise, social or spiritual support—contribute to your ability to resist cold infections and rebound from them quickly.

- Avoid unnecessary ingredients by choosing single over-the-counter remedies that match your symptoms.

- If you do get sick, don't waste energy on self-blame.

- Year by year, build your individual wellness program, your mainstream- and alternative-care team, and your ability to balance health and career demands.

16

Choosing Lozenges

Before you use an over-the-counter throat lozenge, think carefully about why you want to. The most common reasons people use lozenges are to alleviate a hoarse sound, throat pain, and cough. These symptoms often occur together, but not always, and they are relieved by different ingredients.

Some ingredients have side effects you don't want. So it's important to choose the right lozenge for the right purpose. This is especially true if the cough or voice problem lingers after an acute infection—the worst period of misery—has resolved.

Throat lozenges advertised to relieve sore-throat pain or to feel "cool" typically contain menthol, eucalyptus, or benzocaine, which temporarily numb the throat. These lozenges are aromatic, which means you inhale the chemicals as vapors. Unfortunately, the same chemicals that give temporary pain relief also tend to irritate the vocal folds, making the larynx more vulnerable to infection and strain.

You are also more likely to overuse your voice if the "stop, it hurts" signals from your throat are numbed out. Used constantly for more than a few days or during heavy voice usage, these products can make your throat condition and voice worse rather than better.

How to Choose the Ingredients that Suit Your Condition

- If the problem is mostly the sound of your voice, lozenges and sprays won't help. Instead, rest your voice as much as you can, stay hydrated, and use a plain-water (steam) vaporizer in your bedroom or living area for the extra humidity that truly soothes your airway.

- For pain relief related to an acute sore throat associated with a cold, use cooling or numbing lozenges for a few days if necessary. Avoid heavy talking or singing during that time because your vocal cords are swollen and very sensitive to irritation, both from overuse and from the numbing chemicals.

- For a dry-tickly cough, don't use pain-killing lozenges. As soon as they're gone from your mouth, their latent irritation effect may paradoxically increase your desire to cough: a vicious cycle. Steam, fluids, and rest will help much more. Sips of ice-cold water can help "distract" your throat sensations. Nonmedicated lozenges, Life Savers, or hard candies can help stimulate saliva and keep your throat feeling moist; ingredients such as pectin and glycerin are both soothing and safe.

- If your throat hurts for more than a few days, stays hoarse for two weeks, or stays troublesome after other cold symptoms have cleared, don't keep numbing the problem—see a doctor!

Lozenges List

Here are some common lozenges with their active ingredients, as found on the manufacturers' websites. The list in each group is ordered alphabetically by brand name.

Lozenges for lubrication and general throat comfort. No advertised pain relief, no known risk of irritation.

Cold-eeze (zinc)

Halls Breezers (pectin)

Halls Defense (vitamin C, echinacea, zinc)

Hold DM (dextromethorphan, cough suppressant)

Luden's Wild Cherry (pectin)

Smith Brothers (pectin)

Thayers (slippery elm)

Zand Elderberry (zinc)

Zand Herbalozenge (vitamin C, echinacea, zinc)

Lozenges for relief of sore-throat pain. Some risk of vocal-cord irritation. Don't use these for long periods of time.

Bee MD (menthol)

Cepacol (benzocaine and/or menthol)

Cepastat (menthol)

Chloraseptic Sore Throat (benzocaine)

Fisherman's Friend (menthol)

Halls Naturals, Plus, Regular, Sugar Free (menthol)

Luden's Honey Lemon (menthol)

N'Ice (menthol)

Olba's Pastilles (menthol)

Ricola (all) (menthol)

Sucrets (all) (menthol and/or dyclonine)

Throat Discs (anise oil, peppermint oil/menthol)

Vicks (benzocaine, menthol)

This information is provided for educational purposes only. It is not a criticism or endorsement of any product, brand, or remedy, and is not intended to diagnose or treat any medical condition or disease. For more help, talk to a health practitioner or pharmacist who knows your individual needs. If throat pain, cough, or hoarseness last more than two weeks, see a doctor.

Chapter 16 Summary

- Use throat lozenges carefully, for specific needs and discomforts.

- Lozenges with menthol in them are heavily advertised, but often not the best choice.

- Milder, moisturizing lozenges can be found easily if you read the labels.

- Instead of numbing throat pain, rest your voice when it hurts or sounds bad.

17

Using Herbs and Supplements

Chapter 13, "Alternative Medicine," explains why many people, and perhaps especially creative artists, choose nonconventional treatments as part of their approach to health care. Herbs, vitamins, and other supplements are one component of alternative care, and many of my clients ask about them. Although I'm not formally trained in this subject, I try to learn from those who are.

I don't believe that herbs, supplements, and other "alternative" care are inherently good for you compared with doctor-prescribed drugs. Nor do I believe they are inherently bad. These remedies are just different—culturally, commercially, and aesthetically. They may offer genuine health benefits, and because they can be bought without a doctor's oversight, they can offer an appealing feeling of independent self-care and self-management. My own daily regimen includes some of each.

The information offered below comes from recent, respected publications in the field of herbal medicine, with some comments from my personal experience. If something below is listed as uncertain in benefit according to the newest research, but you believe it helps you, thank the plant energy and the very real placebo response for activating your unconscious healing ability. No information here is intended to diagnose or treat any disease, injury, or diagnosed condition in the individual reader. Please consult with a qualified, licensed health-care provider.

Herbal Supplements

Aloe Vera Gel
Benefits: The gel form of aloe vera can be soothing to the stomach and protective against acid reflux.
Caution: The juice form of aloe is made from a "latex" layer of the plant, which has a stronger laxative effect and may cause digestive cramps.

Cayenne Pepper
Benefits: Warming to throat and stomach, cayenne is common in many styles of cooking.
Caution: If heartburn or gastroesophageal reflux disease (GERD) exist, cayenne pepper makes them worse and should be avoided.

Chamomile
Benefits: This herb can be relaxing, can calm anxiety, and can be soothing to the digestion.
Caution: Don't use chamomile you have ragweed allergies.

Echinacea
Benefits: Clinical research studies, taken together, show continuing uncertainty about the benefits of this herb beyond a placebo effect.
Caution: Traditionally described as helping the body resist colds and flu, but Dr. Sahelian reports some cases of extreme allergic reactions to echinacea and advises against its use by people

with auto-immune disorders. Other experts caution against using it for more than two weeks at a time, because its effects on the immune system are so uncertain.

Elderberry
Benefits: Extract or concentrated syrup may shorten the duration of influenza.
Caution: None.

Garlic
Benefits: Ingesting garlic may shorten the duration of colds and flu.
Caution: Any "dose" large enough to have benefit may have socially unacceptable odor.

Ginger
Benefits: Ginger relieves nausea, warms the throat and stomach without aggravating heartburn, can be added to chicken soup, used as tea, and used in many other recipes.
Caution: None.

Ginseng
Benefits: Jennifer Ackerman reports that a specialized product called Cold-FX shows promise in reducing the incidence or duration of colds; research is ongoing.
Caution: Ginseng of any kind is considered unsafe for people taking blood thinners and for pregnant or breast-feeding mothers.

Lemon Balm (Melissa officinalis)
Benefits: A calming herb, lemon balm relieves anxiety such as stage fright
Caution: It may decrease alertness, speed of thought, and reflex reaction time.

Licorice Root
Benefits: Licorice root protects the stomach lining and temporarily soothes the throat.
Caution: Unprocessed forms increase blood pressure, so look for "DGL" formulation.

Marshmallow
Benefits: Gargle or drink tea made from this herb for relief of cough or sore throat. It has a possible mild protective effect on stomach.
Caution: None.

Peppermint
Benefits: Tea can help relieve nasal congestion.
Caution: An active aromatic ingredient (menthol) that is common in throat lozenges (see chapter 16, "Choosing Lozenges"), peppermint is believed to irritate the larynx slightly and may irritate the lungs. Mint can also worsen acid reflux because it relaxes the digestive system, including the valves at the top and bottom of esophagus. Small amounts in toothpaste or mouthwash may be tolerated.

Probiotics
Benefits: Probiotics may help to reduce the seriousness of respiratory infections and keep the digestive system comfortable in cases of acid reflux, used alongside antacid medications.
Caution: Formulations vary in their selection and mix of organisms. You may respond better to one formula than to another, so experiment.

Sage
Benefits: Sage is used as a traditional remedy for sore throats and fever.

Caution: Its strong flavor is difficult as a tea, but it goes well in chicken or vegetable soup.

Tea (black/green)
Benefits: Black tea and green tea relieve some bronchial congestion. Its antioxidant ingredients are considered good for maintaining general health.
Caution: See caffeine discussions in chapter 7, "Drink." Green and white teas are milder than black tea.

Valerian
Benefit: Valerian acts as a relaxing, antianxiety sedative.
Caution: The long-term use of this herb has not been studied. Its strong flavor may be disagreeable, and it may alter dreams.

Vitamin C
Benefits: High doses (several grams per day) may, at best, reduce the duration of colds by about one day.
Caution: There is no evidence that it prevents one from catching a cold. High doses can cause diarrhea.

Zinc
Benefits: Evidence is mixed about zinc's effectiveness in reducing symptoms of the common cold. The placebo effect is especially hard to rule out because of its unmistakably strong flavor.
Caution: Taking zinc does not appear to prevent a person from catching a cold.

Chapter 17 Summary

- Herbal and nutritional remedies can be used alongside conventional medicine, if you're thoughtful about them.

- Herbs may have side effects, just as prescription medicines do, depending on your own body chemistry and the quality of the products.

- If you try multiple remedies at once, it is harder to know which ones truly help you.

- More information can be found in the references listed at the back of this book.

IV

Convention:
Real-World Challenges

The first duty of a man is to speak; that is his chief business in this world; and talk, which is the harmonious speech of two or more, is by far the most accessible of pleasures.

—Robert Louis Stevenson

We are social beings by the voice and through the voice; it seems that the voice stands at the axis of our social bonds, and that voices are the very texture of the social, as well as the intimate kernel of subjectivity.

—Mladen Dolar

The best communications technology is the ear.

—Esther Dyson

18

Telephones and Other Electronics

*Is it a fact, or have I dreamt it—that, by means of
electricity, the world of matter has become a great nerve,
vibrating thousands of miles in a breathless point of time?*
—Nathaniel Hawthorne

When patients come to my office complaining of vocal fatigue, they are often surprised by my questions about their use of the telephone. "But I don't talk loudly at all," they say. "I don't know why it really tires me out."

Or (given that I live near Los Angeles): "Well, I have a long commute, two or three hours altogether, so of course I have to get work done on the phone while I'm driving."

Or: "The only time I have to catch up with my mom/friends/kids is when I'm in the car."

The availability of telephone contact all the time, anywhere, has changed our expectations of how much voice usage is normal. Periods of solitude and time-out buffer zones are no longer built in to the rhythm of a day.

There are so many things to attend to, so many details of life to share, so many people we can reach out to more often. Talking nonstop is now possible, so why wouldn't we do it?

The reasons to be careful—mindful—about telephone use are simple yet paradoxical. At home, with minimal background noise and a mouthpiece up close, the voice is typically used at a low level, in a range of pitch and loudness that feel very small and low effort. Physiologically, this is like driving at the slow end of a gear range—15 mph in a highway gear. The vocal mechanism tires out because there is so little energy in the system.

For this problem, I recommend standing up and moving around to keep the body active and engaged; deliberately using a wider, more animated pitch range; and, of course, sipping water to stay hydrated for any call or series of calls longer than about ten minutes.

My job nowadays has quite a bit of talking on the phone, which can also be anti-good singing, because talking on the phone usually requires a softer tone of voice and lower volume, which means I run the risk of whispering, which is absolute murder on the voice. And my workday is no less than 10 hours a day. So, when I do exercise my voice or sing or both, I do it as correctly as I can.
—Ron Stone

E-mail is far more convenient than the telephone as far as I'm concerned. I'd throw my phone away if I could get away with it.
—Tom Hanks

Cell-phone calls made on the run, whether in the car or during other away-from-home activities, carry the opposite problem: having to talk too loudly. There is usually background noise, you are busy with other tasks while talking and listening, and despite the best cellular technology there are still moments of interference or unexpected dropouts.

Worse, we know that the person on the other end of the conversation is probably embedded in a similar soup of distractions. The ad tagline "Can you here me now?" is effective because of our chronic uncertainty about whether we're getting through. This injects further pressure and strain into the vocal instrument.

People unconsciously compensate for each of these conditions by talking more loudly. When several such environmental factors occur at once, it's common for cell talkers to develop a tense, aggressive speech style that can quickly fatigue or roughen the vocal cords.

What to do? Modify both your behavior and the gear with long-term vocal health and endurance as your goal.

Use the techno-gadgetry that is easiest to hear and easiest on your voice rather than choosing whatever is new, expensive, on sale, or has some other extraneous appeal. Minimize what background noise you can; close the car windows and turn the radio off during calls; step outside of noisy restaurants or away from heavy traffic noise.

Especially if most of your cell use is in the car, be sure that you're wearing your headset on the side that works best for you. On the window side, the earpiece might help block road noise. On the other side, less noise might leak in, helping you and listeners concentrate better. With a headset-free, overhead or integrated car system, you are at even higher risk for shouting, so use this "convenience" with great caution.

Adjusting such ergonomics is only half of the solution, though. You also need to limit the length of your phone calls, alternating with vocal-rest breaks. Don't keep talking just because you can or because you've forgotten how to cope with feeling separate and solitary.

Simply put, you take best care of your voice when you prioritize what needs to be said right now and what you can communicate some other way. Even if you've never thought about this before, you can choose to set limits on your voice time. If your voice feels tired or rough, learn to exchange important information, clarify your most important feelings and relationships, then stop!

Computer Mics, Speech Software, and Other Gizmos

Lo! Men have become the tools of their tools.
—Henry David Thoreau

It would be impossible to cover or anticipate all the technologies that currently exist or will exist by the time you read this book. My main advice is to keep all the rest of this book in mind when using them!

Technology can become so captivating—or frustrating—that we disconnect from our physical senses and lose contact with the fundamental body awareness that I emphasize as the cornerstone of vocal wellness. If I sit at my computer too long, my back gets stiff and my breath and voice suffer.

Clients who use speech-recognition software or otherwise interact vocally with technology throughout the day often have to modify their voices to fit the machines. If this is necessary where you work, use other wellness tools to counteract the gear-imposed limitations. If you have some control over your tools, take it.

A simple example applies as much to singers as to professional talkers: microphone placement. (Microphone stands may soon disappear from music in favor of headsets and body mics, but they'll stay a bit longer on public-speaking podiums.)

Don't duck your head to match a mic that's too low or crane your neck for one that's too high. Sit or stand as you would to perform or speak unamplified, then place the mic.

It may take a few seconds to adjust a stand or podium mic to your best position. This pause is well worth it. If your audience can see, hear, and understand you, they won't remember the brief wait. If they can't listen easily, they'll definitely remember the frustration.

When using any kind of microphone stand, my default mic position is aimed at my chin: close enough to pick up clearly but far enough to avoid the worst consonant popping. Most important, it's slightly below my face and thus easy to see over. Your specifications may differ; the main thing is to figure out what really works for you and take the time to set things up well.

If you're at a computer using a built-in mic or a headset but needing to watch the screen as you talk, take breaks and get up from the desk when you can, to keep your body limber. Some positioning may be inflexible. But the gear is there to serve you, not turn you into a machine.

The newest computer can merely compound, at speed, the oldest problem in the relations between human beings. In the end the communicator will be confronted with the old problem, of what to say and how to say it.
—Edward R. Murrow

Chapter 18 Summary

- Adjust your telephone use with voice protection in mind.

- If telephone use is part of a sedentary job, take breaks to move around, keep your body awake, and stay hydrated.

- Use a varied, animated pitch to keep your vocal cords flexible and avoid getting "stuck" at one level.

- If most of your phone use is on the move, choose quiet places to talk, and shorten calls when you can.

- Avoid long calls or long lists of calls when driving unless you have a superquiet vehicle and empty traffic lanes.

- Be realistic about cumulative voice demands both on and off the phone, and prioritize your talking.

- Choose gear that adjusts to you and your best physical posture rather than just adjusting how you talk to suit a machine.

- Use steam, quiet days, and the other guidelines throughout this book to compensate for heavy demands for talking through electronics.

19

Travel

Another morning comes: I see
Dwindling below me on the plane
The roofs of one more audience
I shall not see again.

—W. H. Auden

I'll view the manners of the town,
Peruse the traders, gaze upon the buildings,
And then return and sleep within mine inn,
For with long travel I am stiff and weary.

—From *The Comedy of Errors*, by William Shakespeare

Travel brings special vocal risks. The better your stamina and vocal health when you leave home, the better you'll survive the rigors of the road. You can also take some protective actions while you travel to counteract the risks.

The biggest challenges I hear about from patients and doctors are staying hydrated, managing unfamiliar food or meal schedules, inadequate or erratic sleep, and simple overuse of the voice because so many events get packed into one tour. I also hear from clients that they were so busy on the tour that didn't notice vocal problems right away. These challenges exist in addition to the pervasive sense of time pressure to meet a schedule that may or may not fit your needs for sleep, vocal rest, and physical exercise.

If money is tight or your travel is managed by agencies, tour managers, or other staff, you may not have ideal control over your working and living conditions. Just be creative, using the guidelines throughout this book to find solutions that fit your travel needs. Check out the "Trains, Planes, and Automobiles" (4/3/11) *VoiceBox* podcast at www.voicebox-media.org for a related discussion.

Hydration

The passenger cabin of an airplane has been described as drier than the Sahara Desert. Some symptoms of jet lag may actually be caused by dehydration. The vocal instrument is especially vulnerable to fatigue without adequate water in the body or moisture in the air, so you need to take extra precautions to keep your airway humidified and your body adequately nourished with fluids.

It used to be simple to recommend that vocal professionals drink plenty of water before, during, and after air travel. Newer security rules make it less convenient to bring beverages with you, so carry an empty bottle along, perhaps with a flavoring packet, and fill it when you can. Or just budget some pocket cash to buy water before you board.

Remember to avoid consuming caffeine or alcoholic drinks in the air, as their diuretic effects will make dehydration worse. Bring herbal tea bags with you and request hot water for brewing.

There are some over-the-counter sprays and gels that help keep the inside of the nose moist. Another tip I've learned from other vocalists is to carry a damp washcloth or handkerchief in a small plastic bag and take it out to breathe through from time to time.

When you land, continue to refill your water bottle and sip frequently. As soon as possible after you arrive where you will be staying, take a long shower and inhale the steam. If you are planning a long trip with a heavy performance schedule, especially in a dry environment, consider taking your facial steamer with you.

> If there's one available, I go to the steam room every day for my voice. I spend half an hour there and then I eat, because I can't eat later than four o'clock.
> Then I go for a soundcheck. That's my day.
> **—Phil Collins**

Reflux on the Road

Travel schedules can disrupt your best intentions to control and diminish acid reflux. But a little planning goes a long way.

If you take reflux medications, talk to your doctor about how to stay on schedule with them as you change time zones and deal with irregular meal schedules. Keep some of your medication with you on the plane, train, or tour bus rather than putting all of it in your heavier luggage. That way, you're prepared for schedule changes or unexpected meals.

Bring extra medication with you in case your travel is extended for several days. And no matter how your eating schedule changes in different time zones or cultures, do your best to avoid eating or drinking heavily right before going to sleep.

Sleep

Simple fatigue can lead to vocal strain over the course of a music tour or business trip. Travel with ear plugs, a light-blocking eye mask, and other comforts that help you sleep soundly while traveling.

Musicians who tour on busses may be in a familiar environment night after night, but not everyone gets a comfortable bunk. Engine and road noise every night, plus bus fumes and environmental smoke, may quickly dissipate the glamour of a tour.

No matter what your mode of transportation, remember that drinking coffee and alcoholic beverages makes it harder to sleep. These substances may seem to provide relief from the inevitable fatigue, disorientation, loneliness, and unexpected difficulties of travel. But they will add fatigue in the long run. Avoid or limit them on the road, and you'll be more likely to get enough sleep—the deepest refreshment of all.

Overuse

A primary reason for travel is to communicate directly with friends, family, business associates, or audiences you don't otherwise see. These are all temptations to overuse your voice.

Don't waste your voice—save it for your performance and most important conversations. Avoid speaking over noise, choose social activities with care, and listen more than you talk. See chapter 20, "Meet, Greet, and Party," for specific help at promotional parties.

Whether you're trying to practice good everyday voice care or are recovering from a vocal problem with recommendations to rest or limit voice use, other people may not understand your needs as easily as they would with a visible injury like a broken bone. Strangers and people who haven't seen you in a while won't necessarily know how to help you.

You may not want to compromise your privacy or professional image by talking about your needs in detail. Nevertheless, while planning your trip, discreetly let key people know that you are paying attention to vocal care and that you have some new personal habits. Then stick to those limits as best you can.

Remember—nonvocalists who consider you a "diva" for protecting yourself just don't understand. They don't need to. And you don't need to argue or react to their ambivalence. Rest, breathe, and do your work.

He who does not understand your silence will probably
not understand your words.
—Elbert Hubbard

Paying Attention

Daily diligence is your best protection against injury. No matter where or how you travel, look for ways to move and stretch your body, breathe easily, stay hydrated, sleep adequately, and rest your voice.

Warm up as attentively as when you are at home, even if there is less time. Use your daily warm-up to measure how well your voice is doing under the circumstances and whether you need to be even more careful, especially if you're on an extended trip.

Consider keeping a travel log or diary about how your voice performs and solutions or strategies that seem most helpful. This will also help you remember problems or questions to discuss with your teacher, doctor, or voice therapist when you get home.

Chapter 19 Summary

- Establish healthy habits when you're not traveling, then build in as much health and safety as you can when planning your trip or tour.

- Plan ahead regarding medications, healthy snacks and meals, and opportunities for physical exercise, sleep, and vocal rest. These efforts may seem unnecessary in the excitement of starting an extended trip, but they are your best endurance strategy.

- The time you devote to your self-care plan will pay you back as the travel days go by.

True Notes from the Road

Musician's Diary, Tuesday, 7 p.m.
Twilight. Drizzle. Been driving all day. Three frustrating hours stuck behind a bad freeway accident has me way behind schedule. Played a coffeehouse last night; tomorrow I've got a radio promo and a full-length concert in the back room of a music store.

I pull off the interstate, fumble for my itinerary and cell phone. Tell the friend who's hosting me that I won't make it for supper. Get out to stretch my legs, then grind down the highway for three or four more hours. I'll keep the radio off for a while, do some breathing exercises and vocalize.

Midnight, at the oasis (finally!)
I found a parking space only a block away from where I'm staying, and lugged my stuff up to my friends' third-floor apartment. Played with their new dog while they briefed me on the schedule for tomorrow. It looks like I'll be able to get some decent sleep and have time for yoga stretches and a solid warm-up between brunch and the radio broadcast. Later, we'll swing by the music store for soundcheck, then back to base camp for a shower, light supper, and performance prep.

Wednesday, 5 p.m.
Still gray and drizzling. Soundcheck introduced me to the mic stand from hell: an aging gooseneck that droops out of position on a whim. Fixing it and finding a buzz-free monitor took longer than I'd planned. So I can't take half an hour to choose my earrings.

Thursday, 10 a.m.
Gig drew well despite the bad weather. The guy at the coffee bar next door donated a thermos of herb tea, and my voice stayed clear. Sold almost as many CDs as I'd hoped, then celebrated (quietly) with the local pals who made it all happen. . . . Now I'm back behind the wheel. Today's distance quota is like that old railroad ballad: 500 miles. Despite my best efforts, I'm definitely more tired than when I left home two weeks ago. If I stay disciplined, I will finish this marathon. But please, no more traffic accidents! I want that in my contract.

—Excerpted from the feature "Planes, Trains, and Vocal Fatigue," by Joanna Cazden, in the August 1998 issue of Electronic Musician *magazine. Read the full article at www. voiceofyourlife.com.*

20

Meet, Greet, and Party

A celebrity is one who is known by many people
he is glad he doesn't know.
—H. L. Mencken

Laryngologists say that many actors don't lose their voices
onstage, where they take natural precautions, but at the
parties afterwards where they throw caution to the wind!
—Patsy Rodenburg

I don't want my fans to love me;
I want them to love themselves.
—Lady Gaga

Both singers and talkers spend two kinds of time in public: formal events, performances, or presentations, where you are allowed to be the main voice user, and less formal events, where everyone talks at once. Whether you're an indie solo artist, a corporate manager launching a new project, or an entourage-surrounded pop star, your official "show" is typically less of a vocal problem than the social hours that surround it.

Onstage or at a speaker's podium, you present something you've practiced. You're probably amplified; your listeners are not. The background noise level is somewhat predictable, somewhat in your control. You're conscious of your role as performer—you've practiced for it—and other people recognize their role as listeners.

As soon as you get offstage, those subtle protections are gone. As you shake hands, sign memorabilia, and make business contacts for the future, you're improvising over multiple conversations in uncontrolled background noise with lots of demands on your attention.

If refreshments are served—especially alcohol—the people around you get even louder, friendlier, and less able to respect your need to protect your voice for the performances yet to come. (They won't be at the next gig; you will.)

In these "meet and greet" situations, I think that people really want your attention and approval, more than they want to hear you talk. People want to share in your celebrity, to feel warmed by your spotlight.

They may praise your work, pitch new projects, ask follow-up questions, and perhaps challenge you with competitive questions. Underneath all of those interactions, their unconscious goal is to rebalance the power relationship created when you were onstage and they were in the audience.

The best way to protect your voice when interacting with your fans is to relax and let them be. Whether you're exhausted, keyed up, or somewhere in between, you can greet people enthusiastically, beam energy back at them, and still not overuse your vocal cords. Smile a lot, ask questions, and let everyone else talk.

Give every man thine ear, but few thy voice.
—From *Hamlet*, by William Shakespeare

Chapter 20 Summary

- Whenever possible, schedule meet-and-greet sessions after your formal presentation, not before.

- Grab a few moments of silent voice rest before you head into the crowd. Inhale through your nose to relax and rehydrate the inner airway, and drink some water to rehydrate your body from the exertion of your performance.

- If you didn't eat much before the show, refuel with a quick private snack so you won't be distracted during the party and won't have to eat as much later on (closer to bedtime).

- Take a position at the edge of the group, not in the middle, and stay as far as possible from the music speakers, bar, hallway, or other loud hot spots. (Just like before you go onstage, scope the room in advance!) A wall behind you helps to reflect your sound, and cuts in half the noise immediately around you.

- Sip water or juice constantly, rather than alcohol or coffee.

- Keep your face and heart open, but your mouth closed.

Knowledge speaks but wisdom listens.
—Jimi Hendrix

21

Trade Shows and Exhibitions

Speech is power: speech is to persuade,
to convert, to compel. It is to bring another
out of his bad sense into your good sense.
—Ralph Waldo Emerson

You can't learn anything new while you're talking,
yet many entrepreneurs seem to never stop. It's a sad
spiral, since the more you talk, the less people really
hear, meaning they don't learn anything either. . . .
Communication doesn't happen unless both parties
practice the art of effective listening.
—Marty Zwilling

Conventions, trade shows, and other high-contact events over multiple days are often at the heart of business. They can also leave you hoarse, even if you don't have one particular onstage presentation to worry about.

You're in public all the time, and you may feel as though you talk nonstop. I hear similar complaints from clients whose jobs involve interviewing people in background noise, shouting over music in a retail setting, or hawking wares at crowded markets.

For special one-shot events, however, the vocal risks go beyond the sheer number of hours you spend talking in an exhibit hall, meetings, business meals and parties, or on the phone. Add background noise, lack of sleep, different food and drink than your body and schedule are used to, and elevated stress as you rush to meet important people, make new connections, and squeeze benefit out of every minute of the event.

Each of these factors can contribute to wear and tear on your vocal cords or keep your body from restoring and refreshing the special cells that make your voice vibrate. When so many risks combine over a single week or weekend, it's no surprise that you come home sounding hoarse, your throat feeling sore, dry, or muscle-achy. Worse, you might lose your voice and handle the last bits of business croaking like an apologetic frog.

Trade-show hoarseness may seem like a badge of honor—if you've used up your voice, surely everyone will believe that you've totally worked the show! But wouldn't it be nice to work that hard and still sound good when it's over? It is possible if you apply to your voice the same strategic planning you depend on for the rest of your business.

At first, it can feel odd to be so conscientious about the communication tool you generally take for granted. The reward will be a stronger, more confident voice that survives through the final hours of the show—just in time to close that last important deal and greet your family when you get home.

No matter what I do for a living, I have a choice between reaching for enlightened options or less enlightened options. And if I consistently reach for the most enlightened options in any circumstance, I am doing my spiritual practice in the context of the world.

—Peter Coyote

More Tips for Trade Shows

Stay hydrated. Keep a water bottle with you; sip and refill it often. Remember that coffee and alcohol are dehydrating, so drink water between those jolting cups of joe, and alternate alcoholic drinks with water or soft drinks.

Take a few minutes every hour not to talk at all. Elevator rides, walks, or taxi rides between venues need not be crammed full of conversation. Instead, collect your thoughts, listen to others, and let your vocal cords recover for the next onslaught. Athletes are allowed to recover between high-stress games, and your voice box will thank you for every brief "time out" you give it.

Hold one-on-ones and small meetings in the quietest corners of the convention site or lobby. Drawing someone aside might take a few extra moments, but it allows both of you to focus on the work at hand rather than on yelling over noise. If this isn't possible every time, even occasional breaks in quieter surroundings will help you manage the vocal marathon.

Avoid big meals late at night. Whether or not you've been diagnosed with acid reflux, your digestion can be upset by heavy, unfamiliar food on top of packed-schedule stress. Business dinners can be just as friendly if you eat lightly, drink more water than wine, and go easy on fatty and spicy foods. You'll sleep better and perhaps have more time for a solid, nutritious breakfast the next day.

Speech Adjustments for Background Noise

When you need to talk over noise—whether at a crowded entertainers' party or in a booming convention hall—instead of being intensely loud, be intensely clear. Talk a little slower to allow listeners extra time to process your message through the distracting din.

Pronounce your consonants carefully. People instinctively read lips when sound gets muddy, so good articulation helps them to see as well as hear your message. Practice this careful speech rate and clarity on sentences you know you'll be repeating a lot as you prepare for the event. Keep your pitch variable and animated, both to keep listeners' interest and to protect your voice. Work with a speech coach for fine-tuning.

Chapter 21 Summary

- Plan ahead for the vocal demands, as well as business demands, of loud social situations.

- Drink more water than alcohol or coffee; eat carefully and get the best sleep you can.

- Take the initiative to meet important contacts in quiet places, at least a few steps away from crowded parties or booming exhibit halls.

- Listen more than you talk.

- Build vocal rest and physical exercise into your travel or tour schedule.

- In any kind of background noise, emphasize intelligibility —being understood—and meaningful communication, more than brute vocal power.

Pretend that every single person you meet has a sign around his or her neck that says, "Make me feel important." Not only will you succeed in sales, you will succeed in life.

—Mary Kay Ash

Do your work, then step back—The only path to serenity.

—From the *Tao Te Ching*, attributed to Laozi

22

Tobacco, Alcohol, and Marijuana

I have no inhibitions about smoking or drinking,
but I think too much of my voice to place it in jeopardy.
I have spent many good years in training and
cultivating it, and I would be foolish to do
anything which might impair or ruin it.
—Jeannette MacDonald

You are the instrument. A guitar player immediately puts
his guitar away or at least keeps it in a special stand and
cleaned off and would not think of pouring alcohol on it
or dragging it through the mud. Horn players polish and
clean the instrument every day. A violin is taken out of its
case only when it is to be played. But the voice
is exposed to all the elements of the environment, 24/7.
Does that mean sacrificing the "party" materials
in order to have a voice? You betcha.
—Ron Stone

Tobacco

C igarette smoking is well known to contribute to serious health problems, including cancer, heart disease, high blood pressure, and emphysema. Now banned in many public places but still common in others as well as in private, tobacco smoke also contains chemicals that damage the cells inside the voice box.

Inhaled smoke is burning hot, which traumatizes the vocal folds with every puff. After just a few months of constant cigarette use, the mucous membranes inside the voice box become yellow-stained from nicotine, just like the fingers that hold the cigarettes.

Over time, exposure to the heat and chemicals in cigarette smoke makes the vocal folds inflamed and swollen with extra fluid as the body tries to protect itself. The voice sounds rough and low pitched.

Just like those in the nose, the passages of the lower airway are lined with mucous membranes and with microscopic hairs called *cilia*. These cells gather and clear germs and debris out of the lungs. Hot chemical smoke paralyzes them, so they can't do their protective job.

As a result, smokers are more likely to get bronchitis and other respiratory illnesses. Frequent, persistent coughing may further damage the vocal folds.

If you wouldn't dance barefoot on a chemical fire, why would you repeatedly pull hot toxic smoke across your vocal cords? The only good answer is that tobacco is highly addictive, cleverly marketed, and tough to break away from.

For the sake of your long-term health and especially for your voice, use any and all available tools, medications, support groups, and online clubs to help you quit smoking. It often takes several tries to extinguish this habit permanently, so if you relapse, don't give up—look for even more support. At the end of this chapter is a list of the health benefits you'll gain after you stop.

> I'm more proud of quitting smoking than of anything else
> I've done in my life, including winning an Oscar.
> **—Christine Lahti**

If you don't smoke but often perform in smoky settings, the other health ideas in this book will help to protect your voice and recover quickly from smoke-related irritation. (That doesn't mean that the other chapters can make up for continuing to smoke! It doesn't work that way.)

While you can't always control work or living environments, the very real health dangers of second-hand smoke are beyond question. Ask people who truly support your vocal development to help keep the air around you clean.

Alcohol

> Alcohol is a good preservative for everything but brains.
> **—Mary Pettibone Poole**

As I've already discussed, drinking alcohol can contribute to both dehydration and acid reflux. Alcohol can also interfere with getting restorative sleep. So please take alcohol seriously as a general risk factor to vocal health. An additional danger is that when you drink you lose good judgment about how much and how loudly you use your voice.

There are some reported health benefits of wine, however, and the risk of physical addiction for alcohol is not quite as high as for tobacco. So I don't think voice users need to be as strict about using alcohol as they should with smoking.

Nevertheless, I worry when a young performer, student, or business speaker casually describes a social life built around clubs and bars, where they have several drinks each night most nights of the week. I advise my clients to stay conservative, stay mindful, and to drink nonalcoholic beverages most of the time.

Mariachi Melancholy

Student question:
My brother sings with a mariachi band at a big restaurant. You know, he has to sing loud over the trumpets and everything. They're onstage for an hour at a time, and they play six sets every night, six nights every week. Now that I'm taking voice lessons, I asked him about his job.

He says that whenever the guys feel their throats hurting, they take a shot of tequila, and then they can do the next set okay, finish the show. Does that really work?

Answer:
Your brother and his friends in the band certainly work hard, and the tequila also works, but only temporarily. Sadly, in the long run, it will probably make their voices worse.

Alcohol, of course, generally reduces pain in the body. The strong sensation of swallowing straight tequila would "distract" from a sore throat, at least for a few minutes. Alcohol may also feel relaxing and may reduce these singers' anxiety about being able to do their job. It might even relax their throats so that singing feels easier. All of these short-term effects are real and will help them get through that show.

Once the last set is over, though, these singers will be at higher risk for vocal problems. Unless each one also drinks a tall glass of water at every set break, they'll get dehydrated, and their voices could get more tired or strained just from that loss of fluid.

Such a singer is very likely to have reflux episodes overnight, which could actively irritate the vocal cords. He might sleep deeply at first, but after a couple of hours, not so well. So there could be a chronic effect of feeling run down and having to push his voice for the next day's show.

Despite feeling tired, dry, or sore-throated, your brother or his friends may socialize more loudly and freely during breaks as the alcohol loosens their social style. Those breaks would otherwise be important times for vocal rest and gentle physical and vocal warm-up exercises.

Finally, there is the risk for alcoholism if someone relies on tequila to medicate his voice like this several nights every week. This risk would be highest among those whose parents also struggle with alcohol or alcoholism, indicating a biological weakness.

Student:

So what can I do to help them? What can I possibly suggest? I have an office job with health insurance, so I can see a doctor when my throat hurts. But these guys don't. They'd have to just go to the county hospital or the emergency room, and they hate it. It's not like seeing a specialist anyway.

Answer:

Perhaps you can help these singers save up to see a throat specialist (laryngologist) and figure out why their throats hurt.

Treat the cause, not the symptom.

Meanwhile, suggest that they sip ice water instead of tequila. Ice water has a mild numbing effect on the throat, and along with generally increased hydration it will help those long performances. Then teach them the straw-kazoo exercise described in chapter 10, "Warming Up the Voice." If you think the band would go for it, I could do a group class sometime and teach them more warm-ups.

Student:

That's a great idea, but these are macho guys. They won't want to listen to a woman. They don't listen to me much at all about anything, but I'll keep trying.

Marijuana

During a typical voice examination, ask a rock singer whether they smoke, and they'll look up with a guarded-yet-mischievous half smile and say, "Well, not tobacco, but . . ." Most pot users have done re-search online or among their friends and learned that marijuana burns hotter than tobacco but has fewer extra chemicals in it. So they'll smoke marijuana using a water pipe or vaporizer, or consume "edible" forms, and figure it's safe enough.

I confess that there have been times in the past when I reached for marijuana for relaxation and pleasure. I believe that weed use is probably less harmful to the body overall than tobacco smoke and lower risk to the voice using the precautions described above.

Nevertheless, I don't think marijuana is anywhere near risk-free, especially for those who use it regularly. It is also still illegal. The mental effects of weed—including the complications of obtaining it and a real risk of psychological addiction—need to be considered along with the physical effects in making your most informed decision about what's best for your voice and voice use.

Consider that throughout this book I emphasize that the voice benefits from clear awareness of mind and body and of their relationship to the feelings you want to communicate. Any chemical that dulls your awareness of your body sensations, that reduces your motivation to practice and exercise, or that otherwise decreases your daily dedication to a healthy lifestyle, is likely to interfere with your vocal development and wellness.

I've seen a few clients who disclosed to me that they use marijuana regularly. Anecdotally, these people shared a tendency to focus better on theory than practice, enjoying the concepts of vocal function more than actually mastering my recommended exercises. They were very pleasant people, but mentally mildly fuzzy no matter the time of day, and they tended not to practice much at home.

I agree with Andrew Weil, MD, that formal research into marijuana's mental effects has many methodological problems and that the chemistry of marijuana seems to interact with powerful placebo effects. From my perspective as an advocate for vocal cords and healthy technique, I'd just ask that you prioritize carefully.

If you find yourself not achieving the vocal goals you've set for yourself, and you feel anxious or resentful about the possibility of giving up weed, you may have a problem with marijuana and may benefit from getting help to stop using it. At the very least, don't take risks with illegal activity, and avoid hot smoke of all kinds.

Chapter 22 Summary

- Despite the romantic mythology, alcohol and other drugs, including cigarettes, are not required for artistic creativity, and they are likely to hurt a long-term career.

- Compared with a life full of smoke, drugs, and alcohol, a healthy lifestyle will give you deeper pleasure in the long run—and a much, much healthier voice.

- If you smoke cigarettes, please do whatever it takes, however long it takes, to quit. If you don't smoke, keep it that way.

- Alcohol can harm your voice in multiple ways; the most immediate risks are dehydration, acid reflux, and less control over your loudness. The greatest long-term risk is true addiction, which hurts much more than your voice. Be careful.

- The risks and benefits of marijuana remain controversial and under investigation. If it is currently part of your lifestyle, protect your throat by using a vaporizer or nonsmoked forms, and get real about its effects on your mental discipline and your progress toward career goals.

- A generally clean-and-sober lifestyle shows the extra care that your voice appreciates and deserves. But don't take my word for it. Be honest with yourself and give it a try.

How Your Body Recovers When You Quit Smoking Cigarettes

- **20 minutes after the last cigarette:** heart rate drops
- **12 hours after the last cigarette:** the carbon monoxide level in the blood drops back to normal
- **2 weeks to 3 months after the last cigarette:** circulation improves and lung function increases
- **1 to 9 months after the last cigarette:** coughing and shortness of breath decrease; cilia (tiny hairlike structures that move mucus out of the lungs) begin to function normally again, increasing the ability to clean out the lungs and thus reduce the risk for lung infection
- **1 year after the last cigarette:** risk of heart disease is decreased in half compared with a smoker's risk
- **5 years after the last cigarette:** risk for having a stroke is the same as a person who never smoked
- **10 years after the last cigarette:** lung-cancer death rate is about half of a smoker's; the risk of cancer of the mouth, throat, esophagus, bladder, cervix, and pancreas decrease as well
- **15 years after the last cigarette:** the risk of heart disease is the same as a person who never smoked

—Adapted from "The Health Benefits of Smoking Cessation: A Report of the Surgeon General," 1990 (http://rtips.cancer.gov/rtips/viewProduct.do?viewMod e=product&productId=189642)

I made a commitment to completely cut out drinking and anything that might hamper me from getting my mind and body together. And the floodgates of goodness have opened upon me, spiritually and financially.

—Denzel Washington

One day I promised God that if he would give me my voice back I would never smoke again. I got three octaves back after quitting.

—Mariah Carey

V

Extension:
Your Vocal Future

Human speech is like a cracked kettle on which we tap
crude rhythms for bears to dance to, while we long to
make music that will melt the stars.
—Gustave Flaubert

The moment we begin to fear the opinions of others and
hesitate to tell the truth that is in us, and from motives of
policy are silent when we should speak, the divine floods
of light and life no longer flow into our souls.
—Elizabeth Cady Stanton

Doing your best at this moment puts you
in the best place for the next moment.
—Oprah Winfrey

23

Training

Methinks thy voice is alter'd; and thou speak'st
In better phrase and matter than thou didst.
—from *King Lear*, by William Shakespeare

I had a really good teacher. This is what made all the
difference. A good teacher will teach you the technique,
but also how to listen to your voice.
—Cecilia Bartoli

While I am grateful to all of my excellent teachers for
the many valuable things they taught me, I had a strong
feeling that there was something which I must know and
which only I could find out for myself.
—Evan Williams

'll never forget my first voice lesson. I was 11 years old, trying out
for a neighborhood children's theater show. The director kindly
asked me to wait after the others left and then walked some dis-

tance away. She turned back to face me and said, "Do you think you could talk louder, without shouting?"

Something flipped on—or flipped over—in my stomach, and I found myself doing exactly what she wanted: talking louder without shouting. I'm still not sure how I did it, or how she got me to experience something so new. The mystery of that moment continues to sustain my passion for the phenomenon of voice.

I've studied since then with singing teachers good and bad, theater teachers clear and confusing, speech pathology professors, and education experts in many related fields. There have been choral and theater directors, acting and movement teachers, body workers, yoga instructors, and clinical supervisors who showed me how to be—or how not to be—effective. I like to borrow Michelangelo's motto *Ancora imparo*, or "I am still learning."

Voice Training Options

There is no substitute for real-time contact with a good individual voice teacher. You can save money by going to group classes, or getting exercises online or on CD/DVD and experimenting on your own. I've listed a few favorite resources at the end of this chapter. But in many ways, vocal technique is learned (and therefore transmitted) nonverbally, through an empathic connection with another, more knowledgeable person's body-mind.

The dangers of this connection are also real. Vocal lore is full of teacher-student relationships that are demeaning, abusive, or simply frustrating. Like everything else about the vocal instrument, voice training is unavoidably personal, even if there is no physical touch or discussion of private topics.

Be thoughtful and self-aware when choosing a voice teacher or working with one assigned to you in a training program. The best teacher for you may not be the one your friends, idols, or family would choose, and the training approach that suits you best may or may not be the most famous or even the most expensive.

Finally, a singing teacher or speech coach should be able to distinguish an untrained voice from a damaged or unhealthy one. So if your teacher advises you to see a doctor, do it! But if an artistic teacher tries to diagnose what's wrong with your voice, or claims that they can "fix you" without a doctor's exam, go to the doctor anyway, then find another teacher.

An ideal teacher will do the following:

- Explain enough but not too much, presenting the lesson so that you, not they, are active most of the time.

- Address individual problems, adapting their method to fit your needs rather than proclaiming that the same approach works for everyone.

- Review homework instructions and answer questions so that you are secure in what and how to practice on your own.

- Make clear when and if they are teaching you fundamental technique as opposed to performance or presentation style and polish.

- Directly or indirectly teach you how to learn, so that you become confident in your own development.

A good teacher or reliable singing colleague can help us achieve [many] things. But if they are doing the monitoring and advising for us, then we do not learn to trust ourselves. . . . So from the very earliest stages of learning, teachers/choral directors need to help students develop these self-monitoring skills—otherwise, students and teachers unconsciously collude in the student developing a dependency on the teacher and diminished self-trust in practice and performance.

I think a teacher is failing if their student says they always sing better in a lesson than anywhere else.

—Alexander Massey

Speech Training, Even for Singers

Having trained and worked in many types of voice use, I recommend speech-oriented voice work as a universal foundation of other vocal development. (I refer to a general concept here, not to the specific "speech-level singing" method taught in pop music by Seth Riggs and his protégés.)

I know that business-speech professionals may not consider taking voice lessons at all. Singers may not think of studying speech. But hear me out.

First, the voice methods taught to actors emphasize the use of the whole body. These approaches to breath technique tend to be clearer and more flexible than those typically offered to singers; the voice develops with spontaneity, authenticity, and a motivation rooted more in personal meaning than in abstract "style." Singing methods, in my experience, increasingly acknowledge these more somatic, text-oriented rehearsal devices, but do not train yet them fully. Whether in rock, acoustic pop, jazz, or classical styles, one may be at risk for an unnecessary confusion, artificiality, or rigidity in voice technique.

Second, many singers use their voices well when they are singing but don't apply the same principles to speech. If you don't know how to avoid strain in everyday conversation, your singing could be at risk. A spoken-voice method will help protect you offstage while adding dimension to your performance voice.

Third, speech-based training is typically available in group classes, which lowers the cost and decreases the sense of vulnerability common to beginners. You learn to observe and sense many other bodies and voices, honing your self-perception in the process.

Finally, the methods currently used by theater-speech trainers have a young, lively tradition that feels fresher to me than classical singing but more practical and specific than what rock and pop teachers typically offer. These methods are not a substitute for musical training, but they offer a powerful set of complementary tools, especially useful to singer-songwriters and others who emphasize lyrics, storytelling, and naturalistic communication.

Theater-oriented training systems are known by the names of the master teachers who created them—Cicely Berry, Catherine Fitzmaurice, Roy Hart, Kristin Linklater, Arthur Lessac, and Patsy Rodenberg. Younger teachers in your area may adapt or combine methods. I have studied Fitzmaurice Voicework most recently, so this is the system I know best. I respect them all.

Developing my speaking voice with Fitzmaurice and other theater classes helped my singing voice as much or more than my formal singing lessons. I highly recommend this general field of study to singers, public speakers, and all voice users who haven't otherwise encountered it.

Online and Recorded Exercises

There are far too many prepackaged singing programs available now to list here—probably a new one is put up every day on YouTube. Listed instead are less-obvious resources: programs for the speaking voice developed by some of the top theater-oriented trainers around. As explained above, I recommend these methods for singers as well as for talkers because of their emphasis on the use of the whole body and on direct, authentic communication.

- Eric Armstrong's website, The VoiceGuy (http://voiceguy. ca/the-warm-up-series), leads you through three series of voice warm-ups plus a speech warm-up.

- David and Rebecca Carey's *Vocal Arts Workbook* comes with its own DVD.

- Kate DeVore and Starr Cookman's *The Voice Book* comes with a warm-up CD. The authors are both speech pathologists, one a singer and the other trained in theater.

- National Theatre Warm-Up: England's National Theatre presents four training sequences—breathing, resonance, opening up the voice, and articulation.

- National Theatre Voice App: Download the above exercises to iTunes. Works on Mac, iPad, and PC.

- Finally, I recommend that all singers become musically literate. If you don't play piano or another instrument, find classes or software in music theory, note reading, ear training, and simple harmony or song structure.

Singers are sometimes stereotyped by other musicians as not knowing how to read music or find their way around a score. Mastering the basics will help you to communicate more easily with other players and to earn their respect. Your career and your confidence will benefit from this investment.

Excellence is an art won by training and habituation. . . .
We are what we repeatedly do.
—Aristotle

Practice isn't about trying to throw ourselves away and become something better. It's about befriending who we are already. The ground of practice is you or me or whoever we are right now, just as we are. That's the ground, that's what we study, that's what we come to know with tremendous curiosity and interest.
—Pema Chodron

Chapter 23 Summary

- Good voice training keeps you sounding natural—like yourself, only better and safer.

- Online and recorded resources can teach you a lot, but the internal, hard-to-describe nature of voice technique makes interacting with a live teacher especially important.

- Try several different teachers if you can; just say at the outset that you'd like a sample lesson, so that everyone's expectations are clear before you begin. Then stay with the one that suits your goals and learning style.

- Most of a voice lesson should be "doing," not listening. If you spend more time with theory or demonstrations than actual muscular practice, your mind may learn a lot but your body and voice will not change.

- A knowledgeable voice teacher recognizes his or her limitations, referring you to medical or rehabilitation colleagues if your voice does not respond to normal training, or to teachers with other specialties if your performance goals change.

- Take occasional workshops or lessons in an unfamiliar style of voice use for a fresh experience of your instrument.

- Both singers and talkers benefit from the voice methods used in theater programs.

24

Intangibles

*A voice that is free, that feels its inherent right to speak,
will have no fear of calling out, whenever
and wherever it is needed.*

—Arthur Lessac

The Voice of Your Life

Creating the sounds of singing or speech unites all the essential elements of life. Using one's voice and being heard by others is an amazing biological act. It is also an important expression of life, freedom, spirituality, individuality, and community.

If your voice is struggling, it may be normal to experience the problem as simultaneously personal and interpersonal, deeply private yet impossible to hide. When my speech-therapy clients lose their voices completely or are advised for medical reasons to rest in silence as much as possible, they are often astounded at how deeply this changes their relationships and their place in the world. Long-lasting,

whole-person-oriented care for the voice may require acknowledge-
ment of the subtler dimensions of its meaning.

When circumstances require us to withhold important truths, to
keep silent when we long to shout for attention or for justice, the
block may be felt physically as a "lump in the throat." But when we
say things that are true, "sing from the heart," or find the courage to
"speak truth to power" as the Quakers put it, the voice may carry its
greatest power and richness of sound.

This is not to imply that vocal problems are "all in your head." If
your voice is suffering from a clearly organic cause—such as medical
side effects of another condition or treatment—voice care may simply include a deeper appreciation for human communication in all its
forms.

But if your voice develops a problem related to usage, consider
whether there is a hidden message, some part of you that is struggling
to be "heard." Paradoxically, vocal rest can be a time for listening to
the "inner voice," allowing unexpected truths to emerge from within.

Wellness in the World

Similarly, when things are going well, a healthy vocal sound indicates
to others that your body, mind, and spirit are balanced, integrated,
vibrant, and expressive. Your voice, like other parts of your individual
nature, is unique in human existence, and its capacity is worth developing and protecting.

Balanced nutrition, exercise, rest, satisfying relationships, and an
authentic, optimistic spirit are good for your overall health and good

for your voice. Let your desire for a healthy voice help motivate you to take good care of your body and mind and to build a life and lifestyle that support and express your unique self.

Chapter 24 Summary

- Like vocal expression, voice care is very personal.

- Resting your voice in silence may allow your "inner voice" to become stronger.

- Learning how to take care of your voice can open a deeper understanding of how your mind, body, and emotions interact.

- As these elements become more balanced and healthy, the sound of your voice will grow and thrive.

Lift every voice and sing till earth and heaven ring,
Ring with the harmonies of liberty.
Let our rejoicing rise high as the listening skies;
Let it resound loud as the rolling sea.
—James Weldon Johnson

He who sings frightens away his ills.
—Miguel Cervantes

References and Suggested Reading

Websites

The Voice of Your Life: Vocal Health Resources for Singers & Speakers
(Joanna Cazden's coaching/therapy site)
www.voiceofyourlife.com

Also referenced in this book are the following websites:

American Speech-Language-Hearing Association
(A professional organization for speech pathologists and audiologists, the site includes consumer information about voice, speech, and hearing problems.)
www.asha.org

Dr. Ray Sahelian, MD
(This site gives detailed information on hundreds of nutritional

supplements, herbal remedies, and health topics from a point of view that integrates alternative and conventional medical care.)
www.raysahelian.com

Fitzmaurice Voicework
(See a calendar of workshops worldwide and a directory of teachers.)
www.fitzmauricevoice.com

The Health Benefits of Smoking Cessation: A Report of the Surgeon General
(This simply-worded 1990 motivational summary shows how health improves after someone quits smoking.)
http://rtips.cancer.gov/rtips/viewProduct.do?viewMode=product&productId=189642

The Modern Vocalist World: Social Media for Singers!
(This social media network of singers and teachers, primarily pop and rock orientated, also has forum discussions that include health topics.)
www.themodernvocalist.com

National Association of Teachers of Singing
(See the teacher directory)
www.nats.org

National Referral Directory
(Laryngology and voice rehabilitation providers, provided by the Johns Hopkins Voice Center at Greater Baltimore Medical Center)
www.gbmc.org/home_voicecenter.cfm?id=1551

Oxford Singing Lessons: Voice Development and the Psychology of Learning and Performance
(This site is the source of quotations from voice teacher Alexander Massey)
www.oxfordsinginglessons.co.uk

VASTA: Voice and Speech Trainers Association
(This site includes an international directory of speech and voice teachers, and an extensive bibliography on voice and speech topics.) *www.vasta.org*

Voice Academy
(This site is a no-cost, self-directed, virtual school built for the vocal health of U.S. teachers.) *www.uiowa.edu/~shcvoice*

The Voice and Swallowing Institute of the New York Eye and Ear Infirmary (This site includes a good description of speech therapy for voice problems)
www.nyee.edu/cfv-therapy.html

The Voice Guy: Voice and Speech for the Professional and Aspiring Actor.
The Warm-Up Series (downloadable warm-ups for the speaking voice, from theater professor Eric Armstrong)
http://voiceguy.ca/the-warm-up-series

Books and Articles on Voice Production, Vocal Health, and Training

Abitbol, J. 2006. *Odyssey of the Voice*. Translated by P. Crossley. San Diego, CA: Plural Publishing Inc.

Barton, R., and R. Dal Vera. 2011. *Voice: Onstage and Off*. 2nd ed. New York, NY: Routledge.

Baxter, M. 1991. *The Rock-N-Roll Singer's Survival Manual*. Milwaukee, WI: Hal Leonard Publishing Corporation.

Boren, M. 2005. *Breathing for Performance: A Guide for Wind and Voice Musicians*. Houston, TX: Powerlung Press.

Carey, D. and R. C. Carey. 2008. *The Vocal Arts Workbook + DVD: A Practical Course for Developing the Expressive Range of Your Voice.* London, UK: Methuen Drama.

DeVore, K. and S. Cookman. 2009. *The Voice Book: Caring For, Protecting, and Improving Your Voice.* Chicago, IL: Chicago Review Press.

Douglas, E. 2004. *The Actor's Voice: Interview with Catherine Fitzmaurice.* Actingnow.com; reposted on Fitzmauricevoice.com.

Eisenson, J. and A. M. Eisenson. 1991. *Voice and Diction: A Program for Improvement.* 6th ed. Upper Saddle River, NJ: Prentice Hall.

Hixon, T. J. 2007. *Respiratory Function in Singing: A Primer for Singers and Singing Teachers.* San Diego, CA: Plural Publishing.

Lamperti, G. B. 1957. *Vocal Wisdom.* Translated from the French and edited by Strongin, L., and W. Brown. New York, NY: Taplinger Publishing Company.

Lessac, A. 1967. *The Use and Training of the Human Voice.* Mountain View, CA: McGraw-Hill.

Linklater, K. 1976. *Freeing the Natural Voice.* Los Angeles, CA: Drama Publishers.

Martin, S. and L. Darnley. 1992. *The Voice Sourcebook.* Milton Keynes, UK: Speechmark, Ltd.

Melton, J. and K. Tom. 2003. *One Voice: Integrating Singing Technique and Theatre Voice Training.* Portsmouth, NH: Heinemann.

Miller, F. E. 2003. *The Voice: Its Production, Care and Preservation.* Whitefish, MT: Kessinger Publishing.

Miller, R. 2003. *Solutions for Singers: Tools for Performers and Teachers.* New York, NY: Oxford University Press.

Morgan, M. 2008. *Constructing the Holistic Actor: Fitzmaurice Voicework.* La Vergne, TN: Lightning Source Inc.

Pinksterboer, H. 2003. *Tipbook Vocals: The Singing Voice.* Milwaukee, WI: Hal Leonard Publications.

Rodenburg, P. 1992. *The Right to Speak.* New York, NY: Routledge.

Thurman, L. and G. Welch, G., co-editors. 2000. *Bodymind & Voice: Foundations of Voice Education.* Rev. ed. Collegevill, MN: The Voicecare Network.

Verdolini, K. 1998. *Guide to Vocology.* Salt Lake City, UT: National Center for Voice and Speech.

Willams, E. 1921. "How I Regained a Lost Voice." In *Great Singers on the Art of Singing: Educational Conferences with Foremost Artists—A Series of Personal Study Talks with the Most Renowned Opera Concert and Oratorio Singers of the Time*, edited by J. E. Cooke. Philadelphia, PA: Theo, Presser.

Conventional and Alternative Health References

Ackerman, J. 2010. *Ah-Choo: The Uncommon Life of Your Common Cold.* New York, NY: Hachette Book Group.

Brostoff, J. and L. Gamlin. 2000. *Asthma: The Complete Guide to Integrative Therapies.* Rochester, VT: Healing Arts Press.

Cazden, J. 2010. "Breathing the Sound." *Whole Life Times* (June/July): 18. Also available at www.blogher.com/yoga-singers.

Gagnon, D. et al. 1990. *Breathe Free: Nutritional and Herbal Care for Your Respiratory System.* Twin Lakes, WI: Lotus Press.

Harrington, A. 2008. *The Cure Within: A History of Mind-Body Medicine.* New York/London: W. W. Norton & Company.

Mayo Clinic. 2007. *Mayo Clinic Book of Alternative Medicine: The New Approach to Using the Best of Natural Therapies and Conventional Medicine.* Fairfax, VA: Time Inc. Home Entertainment.

Murray, M. 1998. *Encyclopedia of Natural Medicine.* 2nd ed. New York, NY: Three Rivers Press.

Phaneuf, H. 2005. *Herbs Demystified: A Scientist Explains How the Most Common Herbal Remedies Really Work.* Boston, MA; Da Capo Press: Marlowe & Company.

Sahelian, R., MD. 2011. *Natural Healing Secrets Newsletter* Vol. 8, No. 6 (June). www.physicianformulas.com.

Schachter, N. 2006. *The Good Doctor's Guide to Colds and Flu.* New York, NY: Harper Torch.

Stibal, V. 2008. *ThetaHealing: Diseases and Disorders.* Ammon, ID: Rolling Thunder Publishing.

Tierra, M. 1988. *Planetary Herbology.* Twin Lakes, WI: Lotus Press.

Van Lysebeth, A. 1983. *Pranayama: The Yoga of Breathing.* London: Unwin Paperbacks.

Weil, A. T., MD. 1983. *Health and Healing.* New York, NY: Houghton Mifflin.

———. 1998. *The Natural Mind: An Investigation of Drugs and the Higher Consciousness.* Rev ed. New York, NY: Mariner Books.

———. 2004. *Natural Health, Natural Medicine: The Complete Guide to Wellness and Self-Care for Optimum Health.* New York, NY: Houghton Mifflin.

Scientific and Technical References

American Speech-Language-Hearing Association. 2005. "The role of the speech-language pathologist, the teacher of singing, and the speaking voice trainer in voice habilitation." Available from www.asha.org.

Boekema, P. J., M. Samsom, and A. J. Smout. 1999. "Effect of coffee on gastro-oesophageal reflux in patients with reflux disease and healthy controls." *European Journal of Gastroenterology & Hepatology* 11(11): 1271–76.

Brazer, S. R., J. E. Onken, and C. B. Dalton, J. W. Smith, and S. S. Schiffman. 1995. "Effect of different coffees on esophageal acid contact time and symptoms in coffee-sensitive subjects." *Physiology & Behavior* Mar;57(3): 563–67.

Brinckmann, J. et al. 2003. "Safety and efficacy of a traditional herbal medicine (Throat Coat) in symptomatic temporary relief of pain in patients with acute pharyngitis: a multicenter, prospective, randomized, double-blinded, placebo-controlled study." *Journal of Alternative and Complementary Medicine* Apr;9(2): 285–298.

Brody, J. E. 2007. "You Are Also What You Drink." *New York Times* (March 27). www.nytimes.com.

Chapman, D. B. et al. 2011. "Adverse effects of long-term proton pump inhibitor use: A review for the otolaryngologist." *Journal of Voice* 25(2): 236–240.

Edgar, J. D. 2007. "Is Singing More Difficult After Eating a Meal?" *Journal of Singing* 63(4): 431–439.

El-Serag, H. B., J. A. Satia, and L. Rabeneck. 2005. "Dietary intake and the risk of gastro-oesophageal reflux disease: A cross-sectional study." *Gut.* 54(1): 11–17.

Ford, C. N. 2005. "Evaluation and management of laryngo-pharyngeal reflux." *JAMA: The Journal of the American Medical Association* Sep 28;294(12): 1534–1540.

Grandjean, A. C., K. J. Reimers, K. E. Bannick, and M. C. Haven. 2000. "The effect of caffeinated, non-caffeinated, caloric, and non-caloric beverages on hydration." *Journal of the American College of Nutrition* Oct;19(5): 591–600.

Hindmarch, I., U. Rigney, N. Stanley, P. Quinlan, J. Rycroft, and J. Lane. 2000. "A naturalistic investigation of the effects of day-long consumption of tea, coffee, and water on alertness, sleep onset and sleep quality." *Psychopharmacology* Apr;149(3): 203–216.

Kaltenbach, T., S. Crockett, and L. B. Gerson. 2006. "Are lifestyle measures effective in patients with gastroesophageal reflux disease? An evidence-based approach." *Archives of Internal Medicine* May 8;166(9): 965–971.

Khan, A. M., S. R. Hashmi, F. Elahi, M. Tariq, and , D.R. Ingrams. 2006. "Laryngopharyngeal reflux: A literature review." *Surgeon* Aug;4(4): 221–225.

Koufman, J. A. 2002. "Laryngopharyngeal reflux is different from classic gastroesophageal reflux disease." *Ear Nose Throat Journal* Sep;81(9 Suppl 2): 7–9.

Leonard, R., and K. Kendall. 2001. "Phonoscopy—A Valuable Tool for Otolaryngologists and Speech-Language Pathologists in the Management of Dysphonic Patients." *The Laryngoscope* 111(10): 1760–1766.

Lipan, M. J., J. S. Reidenberg, and J. T. Laitman. 2006. "Anatomy of reflux: a growing health problem affecting structures of the head and neck." *The Anatomical Record Part B: The New Anatomist* Nov;289(6): 261–270.

Montequin, D. "Actors' Guide to the Respiratory System." Paper presented at the Voice and Speech Trainers Association National Convention, Denver, CO. August 2007.

Nilsson, M., R. Johnsen, W. Ye, K. Hveem, and J. Lagergren. 2004. "Lifestyle related risk factors in the aetiology of gastro-oesophageal reflux." *Gut.* Dec;53(12): 1730–1735.

Riesenhuber, A., M. Boehm, M. Posch, and C. Aufricht. 2006. "Diuretic potential of energy drinks." *Amino Acids* Jul;31(1): 81–83.

Simpson, C. B. "Managing Mucous." Paper presented at the Sixth Annual Sin City Laryngology and Dysphagia Conference, Las Vegas, NV. February 2011.

Stookey, J. D. 1999. "The diuretic effects of alcohol and caffeine and total water intake misclassification." *European Journal of Epidemiology* Feb;15(2): 181–188.

Terry, P., J. Lagergren, A.Wolk, and O. Nyren. 2000. "Reflux-inducing dietary factors and risk of adenocarcinoma of the esophagus and gastric cardia." *Nutrition and Cancer* 38(2): 186–191.

Wendl, B., A. Pfeiffer, C. Pehl, T. Schmidt, and H. Kaess. 1994. "Effect of decaffeination of coffee or tea on gastro-oesophageal reflux." *Alimentary Pharmacology & Therapeutics* Jun;8(3): 283–287.

Related Readings on Voice, Speech, Culture and Mind

Chodron, P. 1996. *Awakening Loving-Kindness*. Boston & London: Shambala.

Dolar, M. 2006. *A Voice and Nothing More*. Cambridge, MA: The MIT Press.

Estés, C. P. 1992. *Women Who Run with the Wolves*. New York, NY: Ballentine Press.

Fitzmaurice, C. 1996. "Breathing Is Meaning," in *The Vocal Vision*. Ed. Marion Hampton. New York, NY: Applause Books.

Hitchens, C. 2011. "Unspoken Truths." *Vanity Fair* (610): 92.

Kabat-Zinn, J. 2006. *Coming to Our Senses: Healing Ourselves and the World Through Mindfulness*. New York, NY: Hyperion Books.

Karpf, A. 2006. *The Human Voice: How This Extraordinary Instrument Reveals Essential Clues about Who We Are*. New York, NY: Bloomsbury Publishing.

Locke, J. L. 1998. *The De-Voicing of Society: Why We Don't Talk to Each Other Anymore*. New York, NY: Simon & Schuster.

Ristad, E. 1982. *A Soprano On Her Head: Right-Side-Up Reflections on Life and Other Performances*. Boulder, CO: Real People Press.

Siegal, D. J. 2010. *Mindsight: The New Science of Personal Transformation*. New York, NY: Bantam Books.

Saraswati, S. C. 1966. *Breath of Life*. New Delhi, India: Motilal Banarsidass Publishers Pvt. Ltd. www.mlbd.com.

Zwilling, M. 2011. "You Never Learn Anything While You Are Talking." huffingtonpost.com/business (posted on June 24).

About the Author

Joanna Cazden, MFA, MS-CCC, is a singer, voice teacher, and speech pathologist who has treated more than 1,000 voice-disordered patients at Cedars-Sinai Medical Center, most of them professional or aspiring artists. Her articles on vocal health and technique have appeared in magazines and periodicals such as *Onstage, Folkworks, Electronic Musician, Whole Life Times,* and *The Voice and Speech Review.* She studied music and drama from childhood and toured the United States as a singer-songwriter in the 1970s and early '80s, recording six solo albums and an ensemble CD with Pete Seeger and others. She holds graduate degrees in both performing theater and communication disorders, is a certified teacher of Fitzmaurice Voicework, and has taught at CalArts and the American Academy of Dramatic Art. Also a longtime student of meditation, yoga, and alternative medicine, Cazden lives in the Los Angeles area with her husband, journalist and musician Scott Wilkinson, with whom she directs a community chorus. Her audio program *Visualizations for Singers,* radio and online interviews, and information on her training services are available at www.voiceofyourlife.com.